FOGSI EEBR 2025

Ethical Evidence-Based Recommendations

Polycystic Ovary Syndrome

Disclaimer

This Ethical Evidence-Based Recommendation (EEBR) document is drafted following a consensus between esteemed FOGSI experts and stakeholders and are based on the scientific evidence available at the time of preparation.

EEBRs should be used for information and educational purposes. They do not replace the need for application of clinical judgment to each individual presentation, or variations based on individual patient and resource setting.

Furthermore, EEBRs do not constitute or imply the endorsement of any of the included technologies, therapies, or techniques by FOGSI.

FOGSI EEBR 2025
Ethical Evidence-Based Recommendations
Polycystic Ovary Syndrome

Editor-in-Chief

Sunita Tandulwadkar
MD (Obs and Gyne) FICS (Gyne-Endoscopy) FICOG
President, FOGSI (2025–2026)
Gynecological Endoscopist and ART & IVF Specialist
Head, Department of Obstetrics and Gynecology
Chief, IVF & Endoscopy Center, Ruby Hall Clinic, Pune
Founder and Medical Director
Solo Clinic IVF—A Center for Excellence in Infertility and Endoscopy, Pune
Founder and Medical Director
Solo Stem Cells—A Stem Cell Research and Application Center, Pune
Founder and Director, Alive Regenerative Wellness, Pune, Maharashtra, India

Editor

Madhuri Patil MD DGO FCPS DFP FICOG
Clinical Director
Department of Reproductive Endocrinology
Dr Patil's Fertility and Endoscopy Clinic
Bengaluru, Karnataka, India
Associate Editor, Fertility and Sterility an official publication of ASRM
Chairperson, ASPIRE SIG Reproductive Endocrinology (2021–2025)
President and Founder Member, Fertility Preservation Society of India (FPSI)
Vice President and Founder Member, The PCOS Society India
Vice President, Indian Society for Assisted Reproduction (ISAR)
Board Member, AE-PCOS Society

Experts

N Sanjeeva Reddy MD DGO
Professor
Department of Reproductive Medicine and Surgery
Sri Ramachandra Medical College and Research Institute
Chennai, Tamil Nadu, India

Sujata Kar MD DNB (Obs and Gyne)
Managing Director
Department of Obstetrics and Gynecology
Kar Clinic and Hospital (KCHPL)
Bhubaneswar, Odisha, India

Convener

Pooja Lodha DNB (Obs and Gyne)
Fellow, Fetal Medicine, FOGSI-FMF UK Certified
Lead Consultant
Department of Fetal Medicine
Ruby Hall Clinic and Bharati Vidyapeeth University and Hospital, Pune
Director, Kangaroo Cradle, Fetal Care Centre
Pune, Maharashtra, India

JAYPEE

JAYPEE BROTHERS MEDICAL PUBLISHERS
The Health Sciences Publisher
New Delhi | London

JAYPEE **Jaypee Brothers Medical Publishers (P) Ltd**

Headquarters
Jaypee Brothers Medical Publishers (P) Ltd
EMCA House, 23/23-B
Ansari Road, Daryaganj
New Delhi 110 002, India
Landline: +91-11-23272143, +91-11-23272703
+91-11-23282021, +91-11-23245672
Email: jaypee@jaypeebrothers.com

Corporate Office
Jaypee Brothers Medical Publishers (P) Ltd
4838/24, Ansari Road, Daryaganj
New Delhi 110 002, India
Phone: +91-11-43574357
Fax: +91-11-43574314
Email: jaypee@jaypeebrothers.com

Overseas Office
JP Medical Ltd.
83, Victoria Street, London
SW1H 0HW (UK)
Phone: +44 20 3170 8910
Fax: +44 (0)20 3008 6180
Email: info@jpmedpub.com

Website: www.jaypeebrothers.com
Website: www.jaypeedigital.com

Inquiries for bulk sales may be solicited at: jaypee@jaypeebrothers.com

FOGSI EEBR 2025—Ethical Evidence-Based Recommendations: Polycystic Ovary Syndrome

First Edition: **2025**

ISBN: 978-93-6616-764-0

Printed in India

Contributors

Aneesha Grover
DNB (Obs and Gyne) MSc (Clinical Embryology) Diploma (Clinical ART)
Senior Consultant
Department of Reproductive Medicine
Nova IVF and Fertility
New Delhi, India

Anushree Devashish Patil
MD DGO
Scientist F, Deputy Director Senior Grade, Head of Division of Clinical Research
In-Charge, ICMR–National Institute of Research in Reproductive and Child Health
Multidisciplinary PCOS Clinic
Division of Clinical Research
ICMR–National Institute for Research in Reproductive and Child Health
Mumbai, Maharashtra, India

Asna Beg Ashraf
MD FICOG
Consultant
Department of Obstetrics and Gynecology
Ujala Medical Center
Lucknow, Uttar Pradesh, India

Chandrika Anand
MD DNB
Director
Department of PCOS
Fortis Hospitals
Bengaluru, Karnataka, India

Danne Shaji Philip
MBBS DNB (Respiratory Medicine)
Junior Consultant
Department of Respiratory Medicine
Excel Care Hospital
Bengaluru, Karnataka, India

Darsana G
MBBS DNB (Respiratory Medicine) Fellowship in Allergy and Allergen Specific Disorders
Associate Consultant
Department of Respiratory Medicine
Excel Care Hospital
Bengaluru, Karnataka, India

Deepti Tandon
MBBS MS (Obs and Gyne) Diploma in Hospital Management
Scientist C
Department of Clinical Research
ICMR–National Institute of Research in Reproductive and Child Health
Mumbai, Maharashtra, India

Madhuri Patil MD DGO FCPS DFP FICOG
Clinical Director
Department of Reproductive Endocrinology
Dr Patil's Fertility and Endoscopy Clinic
Bengaluru, Karnataka, India
Associate Editor, Fertility and Sterility an official publication of ASRM
Chairperson, ASPIRE SIG Reproductive Endocrinology (2021–2025)
President and Founder Member, Fertility Preservation Society of India (FPSI)
Vice President and Founder Member The PCOS Society India
Vice President, Indian Society for Assisted Reproduction (ISAR)
Board Member, AE-PCOS Society

Manish R Pandya
MD FICOG FICMH PhD
Professor and Head
Department of Obstetrics and Gynecology
Mahavir Hospital and Manish IVF Center
Surendranagar, Gujarat, India

Mohammad Noor-A-Alam
MBBS FCPS FRCS FACS
Former Unit Head
Department of Surgery
Bangladesh Institute of Research and Rehabilitation of Diabetes, Endocrine and Metabolic Disorders (BIRDEM) and Ibrahim Medical College (IMC)
Dhaka, Bangladesh

N Sanjeeva Reddy MD DGO
Professor
Department of Reproductive Medicine and Surgery
Sri Ramachandra Medical College and Research Institute
Chennai, Tamil Nadu, India

Nagesh NS MS FSGE DNB
Professor, Surgical Gastroenterology
Director, IGOT
Department of Gastroenterology Sciences and Organ Transplant
Institute of Gastroenterology Sciences and Organ Transplant
Bengaluru, Karnataka, India

Nehal Manish Pandya MD DVD
Professor and Head
Department of Dermatology
Mahavir Hospital and Manish IVF Center
Surendranagar, Gujarat, India

Nupoor Rajendra Limaye
MPH Certification in Digital Health MBA HAHCM BHMS
Senior Research Fellow
Division of Clinical Research
ICMR–National Institute for Research in Reproductive and Child Health
Mumbai, Maharashtra, India

Pratik Tambe
MD FICOG FICRM FICMCH FIAOG
ART Consultant
Gynec Endoscopic Surgeon
Department of Obstetrics and Gynecology, Reproductive Medicine
Gynec Endoscopic Surgery
High-risk Pregnancy
Ashirwad IVF
Mumbai, Maharashtra, India
Governing Council Member
ICOG and ICRM
Managing Committee Member
MOGS, ISAR, MSR
Past Chair, FOGSI and AMOGS
Endocrinology Committees

Radha Vembu
MBBS DGO DNB PhD
Professor and Head
Department of Reproductive Medicine and Surgery
Sri Ramachandra Medical College and Research Institute
Chennai, Tamil Nadu, India

Rajesh Pendlimari
MS FSGE (Surgical Gastroenterology)
Consultant
Department of Surgical Gastroenterology
Manipal Hospitals
Bengaluru, Karnataka, India

Rajsekhar Nayak
MS (General Surgery) FRCS (Edinburgh) FRCS (Glasgow)
Consultant Surgeon
Department of General Surgery
Gunasheela Surgical and Maternity Hospital
Bengaluru, Karnataka, India

Rakhi Singh
MBBS DGO DRM (Germany) DPE (Germany) FICOG FIAOG
Director
Abalone Clinic and IVF Center
Noida, Uttar Pradesh, India
President, Noida Obstetrics and Gynaecological Society
Governing Council Member, ICOG
Vice Chairman, UP State ISAR
Peer Reviewer, JOGI
Chairperson, Endocrinology Committee of FOGSI (2020–2023)

Rutvi Manish Pandya MD DNB
Private Practitioner
Department of Dermatology
Mahavir Hospital and Manish IVF Center
Surendranagar, Gujarat, India

Sharmin Abbasi
FCPS MCPS FACS MBBS FART MSc
Fertility Specialist and Associate Professor
Department of Obstetrics and Gynecology
Anwer Khan Modern Medical College Hospital
Dhaka, Bangladesh, India

Shefali Bhardwaj PhD (Food Science)
Founder and Chief Nutritionist
Department of Nutrition
Meraaki Wellness
Navi Mumbai, Maharashtra, India

Shilpa Joshi MSc RD
Consultant Dietitian and Diabetes Educator
Mumbai Diet and Health Centre
Pune, Maharashtra, India

Smitha Moorthy
MD DGO
Consultant
Department of Obstetrics and Gynecology
Sanjeevani Hospital
Thane, Maharashtra, India

Sonia Malik
DGO MD FICOG
Chief Clinical Mentor
Department of IVF and Infertility
NOVA IVF and Infertility
New Delhi, India

Sudhaa Sharma
MD FICOG FICMCH FIMSA FRCP (Edinburgh) FIMA-AMS FIMS MAMS
Former Professor
Department of Obstetrics and Gynecology
Government Medical College, Jammu
Consultant, Madaan Hospital and Research Centre
Jammu, Jammu and Kashmir, India
Vice President, IMS
Honorary Professor, IMA
Managing Committee Member
PCOS Society of India
Editor-in-Chief
JMH (2016–2018)
Member, National Advisory Board and Journal Committee JOGI (2006–2011)

Sujata Kar
MD DNB (Obs and Gyne)
Managing Director
Department of Obstetrics and Gynecology
Kar Clinic and Hospital (KCHPL)
Bhubaneswar, Odisha, India

Suma P Kumar
MRCP MD CCST EX MBA PGDMLE
Consultant Pulmonologist and
Medical Director
Department of Pulmonology and
Sleep Medicine
Excel Care Hospital
Bengaluru, Karnataka, India

Sunita Tandulwadkar
MD (Obs and Gyne) FICS (Gyne-Endoscopy)
FICOG
President, FOGSI (2025–2026)
Gynecological Endoscopist and
ART & IVF Specialist
Head, Department of Obstetrics and
Gynecology
Chief, IVF & Endoscopy Center
Ruby Hall Clinic, Pune
Founder and Medical Director
Solo Clinic IVF—A Center for Excellence
in Infertility and Endoscopy, Pune
Founder and Medical Director
Solo Stem Cells—A Stem Cell Research
and Application Center, Pune
Founder and Director
Alive Regenerative Wellness
Pune, Maharashtra, India

Uday Thanawala
MD DGO FCPS DNB FICOG
Consultant, Obstetrics and Gynecologist
Thanawala Maternity Home and
IVF Centre
Navi Mumbai, Maharashtra, India

Ulka A Natu
MD DGO Embryologist (ISAR Certified)
Advanced Diploma in Yogic Sciences
(University of Mumbai) Diploma in Yoga
Education (Government Approved)
Vice Chairperson, Assessment
Committee, Yoga Certification Board
Ministry of AYUSH, New Delhi Member,
Ethics Committee, Yoga Mimamsa
Scientific Journal, Kaivalyadhama
(Government of India), Lonavala
Director, Department of Obstetrics and
Gynecology, Nest Hospital
Thane, Maharashtra, India

Urmila Nischal MBBS MD (Dermatology)
Director
Department of Dermatology
Nirmal Skin and Hair Clinic
Vijayanagar, Karnataka, India

Vageesh Ayyar Subramanyam
MBBS MD DM DNB MNAMS
Professor
Department of Endocrinology
St John's Medical College and Hospital
Bengaluru, Karnataka, India

Vibhuti Rao BAMS MSc (Yoga) MPH
PhD Scholar
NICM Health Research Institute
Western Sydney University
Penrith, NSW, Australia

Preface

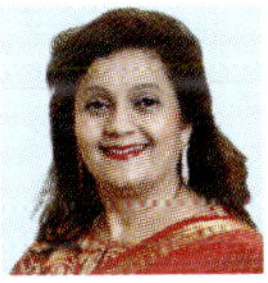

Editor-in-Chief
Sunita Tandulwadkar

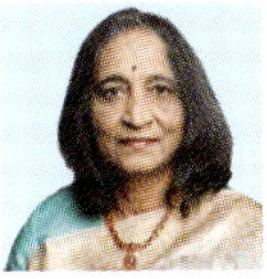

Editor
Madhuri Patil

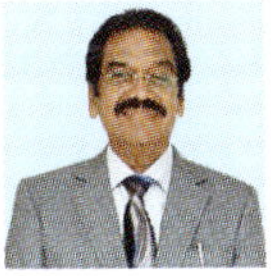

Expert
N Sanjeeva Reddy

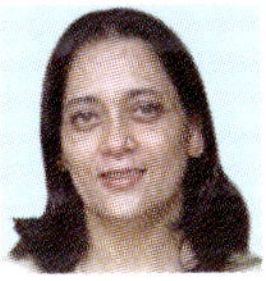

Expert
Sujata Kar

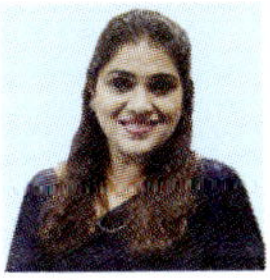

Convener
Pooja Lodha

In the ever-evolving landscape of women's health, it is critical that we remain rooted in ethical and evidence-based practices to guide patient care effectively and responsibly. As the President of the Federation of Obstetric and Gynaecological Societies of India (FOGSI) 2025, I am honored to present this pioneering work, a testament to our commitment to advancing gynecological and obstetric care within India. This book is the outcome of our concerted efforts to create a resource grounded in robust, ethically sound, and evidence-based recommendations that address unique challenges faced by Indian practitioners and their patients.

Globally, esteemed organizations such as the International Federation of Gynecology and Obstetrics (FIGO), American Society for Reproductive Medicine (ASRM), European Society of Human Reproduction and Embryology (ESHRE), and Royal College of Obstetricians and Gynaecologists (RCOG), and other leading societies regularly release recommendations informed by comprehensive research and expert consensus. However, India has long needed its own consolidated guidelines—ones that reflect not only the scientific rigor but also the cultural and social context of our nation. This book represents an initiative to bridge that gap, providing practitioners with authoritative guidelines tailored to our own healthcare environment.

The chapters span a broad spectrum of topics, covering everything from the foundational aspects of prevalence and diagnosis to specialized areas such as lean versus obese polycystic ovarian syndrome (PCOS), mental health screening, and lifestyle management. Expert insights on diet, exercise, pharmacotherapy, and advanced interventions such as bariatric surgery and sleep management are detailed here, helping to address both the fertility and nonfertility aspects of PCOS. Each section is meticulously crafted by respected leaders in their respective fields, who have drawn upon their wealth of knowledge and clinical experience to provide nuanced, practical guidance.

We are deeply grateful to the exceptional team of contributors who have dedicated their time, expertise, and passion to this project. It is our hope that this book will serve as an invaluable resource for gynecologists, bringing clarity and confidence to clinical decisions while uplifting the standards of women's health in India. Together, let us strive to transform these guidelines into everyday practice, benefiting countless women and setting a new standard for ethical, patient-centered care.

We invite you to explore these recommendations and take them forward into your practice, joining us in our mission to shape a healthier and more informed future for women across India.

Contents

Introduction 1

1. **Definition, Prevalence, Diagnosis and Screening of Polycystic Ovarian Syndrome** 59
   Chandrika Anand

2. **Lean versus Obese Polycystic Ovarian Syndrome** 73
   Vageesh Ayyar S, Madhuri Patil

3. **Screening and Management of Mental Health in Polycystic Ovary Syndrome** 84
   Uday Thanawala, Madhuri Patil

4. **Lifestyle Management** 92
   4.1 Diet and Nutrition 92
   Shilpa Joshi, Shefali Bhardwaj
   4.2 Exercise and Yoga 97
   Ulka A Natu, Vibhuti Rao, Smitha Moorthy
   4.3 Behavioral Strategies for Polycystic Ovary Syndrome 105
   Rutvi Manish Pandya, Nehal Manish Pandya, Manish R Pandya

5. **Management of Nonfertility Signs and Symptoms** 111
   5.1 Cosmetic Measures 111
   Urmila Nischal
   5.2 Pharmacotherapy 121
   Rakhi Singh
   5.3 Role of Antiobesity Drugs in Adolescents and Adult Women with PCOS 132
   Pratik Tambe
   5.4 Role of Bariatric Surgery in PCOS 140
   Rajsekhar Nayak, Rajesh Pendlimari, Nagesh NS
   5.5 Common Sleep Disorders in Polycystic Ovary Syndrome 148
   Suma P Kumar, Darsana G, Danne Shaji Philip

6. **Screening and Management for Infertility till Intrauterine Insemination** 158
   Sonia Malik, Aneesha Grover

7. **Role of ART in PCOS: Increasing Efficiency and Reducing Complications** 166
   N Sanjeeva Reddy, Radha Vembu

8. Pregnancy Outcome in Women with Polycystic Ovarian Syndrome 178
Sharmin Abbasi, Mohammad Noor-A-Alam

9. Long-term Health Implications and Comorbidities of PCOS 185
Sudhaa Sharma, Asna Beg Ashraf

10. Patient's Education, Counseling, and Support Groups in Polycystic Ovary Syndrome 199
Anushree Devashish Patil, Deepti Tandon, Nupoor Rajendra Limaye

Introduction

ABSTRACT

Aim: To disseminate evidence-based recommendations for diagnosis, assessment and treatment of PCOS at various stages of life to improve the quality of life.

Participants: Healthcare professionals from different specialities took part in the formulation of these recommendations. The authors and experts for the formulation of these guidelines included gynaecologists, obstetricians, reproductive endocrinologists, endocrinologists, dermatologists and psychology, dietetics, exercise physiology, sleep, and bariatric/metabolic surgery experts.

Evidence: The recommendations involved extensive evidence synthesis and the Grading of Recommendations for writing various chapters by the experts after going through different meta-analyses and the international PCOS guidelines.

Process: Once each chapter with the recommendations was received, the experts studied them and gave suggestions. Once corrections were completed, brainstorming was done by the editor and experts before the final draft was prepared.

What the recommendations do not address?: The evidence used is mostly from international data and not Indian data. Moreover, these recommendations cannot provide full safety and usage information on pharmacological and surgical interventions. We need to modify some of the evidence in the Indian context.

CONCLUSIONS

These recommendations aim to educate the healthcare professionals dealing with adolescent and adult women with PCOS to deliver high-quality, evidence-based assessment and management. These recommendations not only aim at medical and surgical treatment but also at lifestyle modification, which is an important component of PCOS management. We have also included counselling and cognitive therapy, which every clinician should be aware off.

Keywords: PCOS, Adolescence, Diagnosis, hyperandrogenaemia, menstrual irregularity, polycystic ovarian morphology, hyperinsulinemia

Clinical Questions for the Recommendations

1. Definition, Prevalence, Diagnosis and Screening of Polycystic Ovarian Syndrome

1.1. What is the prevalence of PCOS in Adolescents and Adults?
1.2. Is there an ethnic variation in the prevalence of PCOS?
1.3. Criteria for Diagnosis of PCOS—NIH, Rotterdam, AE-PCOS Society, International guidelines on PCOS 2023
1.4. What is new in the diagnosis of PCOS—Role of AMH and ultrasound in PCOS?
1.5. What criteria indicate ovulatory dysfunction in adolescents?
1.6. Can the adult criteria for diagnosis of PCOS be used in adolescent?
1.7. What are the diagnostic criteria for diagnosis of PCOS in perimenopausal and postmenopausal women?
1.8. What are the screening tests and clinical signs for cardiovascular risk?
1.9. What are the screening test and clinical signs of insulin resistance?
1.10. What is the risk in relatives?

2. Lean versus Obese Polycystic Ovarian Syndrome

2.1. What are nutritional and environmental influences throughout the life course and the perpetuation of the transgenerational inheritance of PCOS?
2.2. Why are women with PCOS at increased risk of weight gain and Central Obesity?
2.3. How important is visceral obesity in pathogenesis and clinical manifestation of PCOS?
2.4. Is lean PCOS also obese and why?
2.5. Why are South Asians more prone to insulin resistance?
2.6. What are the similarities and differences between lean and obese PCOS?
2.7. Is obesity associated with greater reproductive dysfunction?
2.8. What is the treatment for lean and obese PCOS?

3. Screening and Management of Mental Health in Polycystic Ovary Syndrome

3.1. What is the prevalence and severity of reduced quality of life?
3.2. What is the prevalence and severity of anxiety and depression?
3.3. What is the prevalence and severity of body image distress?
3.4. What is the prevalence and severity of psychosexual dysfunction?
3.5. What is the prevalence and severity of eating disorders?
3.6. What are the different psychological and therapeutic options that can be offered for the management and support of depression and/or anxiety or disordered eating?

4. Lifestyle Management

4.1. Diet and Nutrition

4.1.1. Are lifestyle interventions effective for improving anthropometric, metabolic, reproductive, fertility, quality of life, and emotional well-being outcomes?

4.1.2. What are the dietary interventions that are effective for improving anthropometric, metabolic, reproductive, fertility, quality of life, and emotional well-being outcomes?

4.1.3. How would you counsel the women with PCOS regarding diet for maintaining the weight?

4.1.4. Barriers to weight loss?

4.2. Exercise and Yoga

4.2.1. What are the components one needs to look at when recommending exercise and yoga to women with PCOS?

4.2.2. Are exercise interventions effective for improving anthropometric, metabolic, reproductive, fertility, quality of life, and emotional well-being outcomes?

4.2.3. Is exercise also important in Lean PCOS?

4.2.4. What exercise would you advise for obese and lean PCOS?

4.2.5. How would you counsel women with PCOS regarding Exercise and Yoga for maintaining weight?

4.2.6. What are the barriers to weight loss?

4.3. Behavioral Strategies for Polycystic Ovary Syndrome

4.3.1. What is the effect of PCOS on the psychological well-being and personality of women?

4.3.2. Can behavior modification interventions aid in the management of PCOS?

4.3.3. What is the utility of mindfulness programs in managing PCOS?

4.3.4. What is the role of cognitive behavioral therapy in the management of PCOS?

4.3.5. What is the consensus regarding use of traditional, complementary, and integrative medicine (TCIM) in PCOS?

5. Management of Nonfertility Signs and Symptoms

5.1. Cosmetic Measures

5.1.1. What is the treatment for acne?

5.1.2. What is the treatment for Hirsutism?

5.1.3. What is the treatment for acanthosis nigricans?

5.1.4. What is the treatment for female pattern hair loss?

5.1.5. How effective are cosmetic procedures?

5.2. Pharmacotherapy

5.2.1. What is the role of combined oral contraceptives (COCP)?

5.2.2. Which is the most effective and safest COCP available and how long should they be continued?

5.2.3. What precautions one needs to take when prescribing COCP in adolescents and adults?

5.2.4. What is the role of Insulin sensitizers (metformin and myoinositols) and should all women with PCOS be given insulin sensitizers?

5.2.5. How long to continue Insulin sensitizers in adolescents and adults?

5.2.6. Is combination therapy of COCP and metformin more beneficial?

5.2.7. What is the role of antiandrogens and which group of women benefit from antiandrogen therapy?

5.2.8. Should antiandrogens be used in combination with other drugs to be more effective?

5.3. Role of Antiobesity Drugs in Adolescents and Adult Women with PCOS

5.3.1. What are antiobesity drugs used for weight reduction and which of them are available in India?

5.3.2. Are antiobesity medications effective as per the evidence from large clinical trials, systematic reviews and meta-analyses?

5.3.3. What are the advantages and disadvantages of the antiobesity agents currently available?

5.3.4. What are the contraindications for using antiobesity medicine?

5.3.5. How long should the antiobesity drugs be administered?

5.4. Role of Bariatric Surgery in PCOS

5.4.1. Is bariatric/metabolic surgery effective for the management of hormonal and clinical PCOS features and weight?

5.4.2. What are the indications for bariatric Surgery in adolescents and adults?

5.4.3. What are the maternal and fetal complications of bariatric surgery?

5.4.4. Can bariatric surgery influence the fertility and pregnancy outcome?

5.5. Common Sleep Disorders in Polycystic Ovary Syndrome

5.5.1. What are the PCOS effects on sleep?

5.5.2. What is the pathophysiology of sleep disorders?

5.5.3. What is the prevalence, evaluation and treatment options for snoring and OSA in PCOS?

5.5.4. How to evaluate and treat Insomnia in PCOS?

5.5.5. What is the management of Restless legs (RLS, Willis–Ekbom Disease) in PCOS?

6. Screening and Management for Infertility till Intrauterine Insemination

6.1. What are the preconception risk factors associated with poor or negative fertility outcomes?

6.2. Is it necessary to confirm that patient is anovulatory before starting any treatment?91
6.3. What test would you do before inducing ovulation?
6.4. Which oral ovulogens will you use and why?
6.5. How will you manage resistance to oral ovulogens?

7. Role of ART in PCOS: Increasing Efficiency and Reducing Complications

7.1. What are the indications for ART in women with PCOS?
7.2. What is the COS protocol of choice?
7.3. How will you prevent OHSS in women with PCOS?
7.4. How will you manage OHSS?
7.5. Is in vitro maturation (IVM) of oocytes treatment of choice in women with PCOS?
7.6. Should metformin be used in all patients undergoing ART?
7.7. How important is lifestyle modification in patients who need ART? What is the evidence?
7.8. How to prevent complications in ART?
7.9. What is the role of freeze all in PCOS women undergoing ART?
7.10. How will you prepare the endometrium for FET?

8. Pregnancy Outcome in Women with Polycystic Ovarian Syndrome

8.1. Are women with PCOS at increased risk of adverse pregnancy outcomes and why?
8.2. What risks have been associated with pregnancy in women with PCOS and how do you prevent them?
8.3. Should Insulin sensitizers be given prophylactically to prevent complications of pregnancy?
8.4. How obesity adds to the complications in pregnancy?

9. Long-term Health Implications and Comorbidities of PCOS

9.1. What is the prevalence of long-term health implications and comorbidities?
9.2. Impaired glucose tolerance and type 2 diabetes—prevention, diagnosis, and management?
9.3. How to prevent, diagnose and manage cardiovascular risks?
9.4. What are the criteria to diagnose metabolic syndrome?
9.5. Does the incidence of gynecological malignancies (endometrium, ovaries, and breast) increase in PCOS?
9.6. How to prevent cancer risk in women with PCOS?
9.7. How do you manage endometrial cancer conservatively?
9.8. Is there an increased risk of inflammation in PCOS?
9.9. What is the prevalence, diagnosis and management of NAFLD and NASH in women with PCOS?
9.10. How will you prevent the occurrence of late sequelae in PCOS?

10. Patient's Education, Counseling, and Support Groups in Polycystic Ovary Syndrome

10.1. What are the characteristics of available models of care implemented in PCOS clinics or services?
10.2. How can we best support women to navigate the impact of PCOS on family and
10.3. What are the key challenges for those with PCOS when interacting with healthcare professionals about PCOS and related features?
10.4. How important are support groups and how do they function?
10.5. Is a questionnaire necessary before counseling?
10.6. Who should counsel women with PCOS?
10.7. Should the counseling be individual or in a group?
10.8. Is patient's education an important aspect in managing PCOS?

Quality of Evidence

Quality of evidence	*Interpretation*
Strong quality of evidence	Evidence from at least one large randomised, controlled trial of good methodological quality (low potential for bias) or meta-analyses of well conducted randomised trials without heterogeneity
Moderate quality of evidence	Small randomised trials or large randomised trials with a suspicion of bias (lower methodological quality) or meta-analyses of such trials or of trials with demonstrated heterogeneity
Low quality of evidence	Prospective cohort studies
Clinical practice points	Evidence not sought. A practice point has been made by the guideline development group where important issues arose from discussion of evidence-based or clinical consensus recommendations.

Recommendation Summary

No.	*Question for recommendation*	*Recommendation*	*Quality of evidence*
1.	**Definition, Prevalence, Diagnosis and Screening of Polycystic Ovarian Syndrome**		
1.1.	**What is the prevalence of PCOS in Adolescents and Adults?**	1.1.1. As the Global and Indian prevalence of PCOS has increased, adults and adolescents suspected to have PCOS should have a diagnostic assessment in accordance with the diagnostic algorithm published by international guidelines.	Moderate quality of evidence
		1.1.2. A timely diagnosis of PCOS in symptomatic adolescent girls is important for the initiation of appropriate screening and treatment.	Strong quality of evidence
1.2.	**Is there an ethnic variation in the prevalence of PCOS?**	1.2.1. There is an ethnic variation in the prevalence as well as clinical presentation and metabolic consequences of PCOS.	Strong quality of evidence
1.3.	**Criteria for Diagnosis of PCOS—NIH, Rotterdam, AE-PCOS Society, International guidelines on PCOS 2023**	1.3.1. In adult women, it is recommended that a diagnosis of PCOS be made using the modified Rotterdam criteria, meeting two of the following three conditions: I. Androgen excess: a. *Clinical:* Persistent acne, hirsutism (A modified Ferriman–Gallwey score of ≥4 to ≥8), female pattern hair loss. Hirsutism should be considered as a strong predictor of hyperandrogenism and PCOS in adults. Acne and alopecia could be considered as being weaker predictors of hyperandrogenism. b. *Biochemical:* • Elevated total or free testosterone, or calculated indices of free testosterone [Free androgen Index (FAI), bioavailable testosterone (BioT)]. • DHEAS and ANSD can be considered	Strong quality of evidence

Contd...

Contd...

No.	***Question for recommendation***	***Recommendation***	***Quality of evidence***
		II. Ovulatory dysfunction: Oligo-amenorrhea (cycles >35 days apart or <8 menses a year). If highly suspicious for PCOS, but does not have oligo-amenorrhea, consider serum progesterone or luteinizing hormone (LH) assessment	
		III. Polycystic ovary morphology (PCOM) on ultrasound using the new criteria: Follicle number per ovary (FNPO) ≥20 in at least one ovary, follicle number per section (FNPS) ≥10 in at least one ovary or ovarian volume (OV) ≥10 mL. If using the transabdominal approach for USG only volume needs to be reported. The number of follicles is best reported only at a transvaginal scan with a transducer frequency ≥8 MHz	
1.4.	**What is new in the diagnosis of PCOS—Role of AMH and ultrasound in PCOS?**	1.4.1. Serum AMH could be used for defining PCOM in adult women as an alternative to pelvic ultrasound but should not be used as a single test for the diagnosis of PCOS and should not be used in adolescents for diagnosis.	Moderate quality of evidence
		1.4.2. AMH level is not necessary for PCOS diagnosis in patients with irregular menstrual cycles and hyperandrogenism.	Moderate quality of evidence
		1.4.3. Age, BMI, use of hormonal contraception, menstrual cycle day and method of assay influence AMH levels.	Clinical practice point
		1.4.4. Follicle number per ovary (FNPO) of ≥20, follicle number per cross-section (FNPS) of ≥10 and ovarian volume (OV) of ≥10 mL should be considered accurate ultrasound markers for PCOM in adults. Transvaginal ultrasound is more accurate than transabdominal ultrasound.	Strong quality of evidence

Contd...

Contd...

No.	***Question for recommendation***	***Recommendation***	***Quality of evidence***
		1.4.5. There are no definitive criteria to define polycystic ovary morphology (PCOM) on ultrasound in adolescents, hence it is not recommended in adolescents.	Clinical practice points
		1.4.6. Either serum AMH or ultrasound may be used to define PCOM; however, both tests should not be performed to limit overdiagnosis.	Clinical practice points
1.5.	**What criteria indicate ovulatory dysfunction in adolescents?**	1.5.1. Irregular cycle and ovulatory dysfunction a. 1 to <3 years postmenarche: <21 or >45 days. b. 3 years postmenarche to perimenopause: <21 or >35 days or <8 cycles per year. c. 1 year postmenarche >90 days for any one cycle. d. Primary amenorrhea by age of 15 years or >3 years postthelarche (breast development).	Strong quality of evidence
		1.5.2. In adolescents, one needs to identify the optimal timing of assessing PCOM which is physiological at that time.	Clinical practice point
		1.5.3. For adolescents who have features of PCOS, but do not meet all three diagnostic criteria, an "increased risk" could be considered and reassessment advised at or before full reproductive maturity, 8 years postmenarche.	Clinical practice point
1.6.	**Can the adult criteria for diagnosis of PCOS be used in adolescent?**	1.6.1. A persistent observation of oligo-/amenorrhea beyond 2 years of menarche with either clinical or biochemical hyperandrogenism is a diagnostic criterion of PCOS in adolescents.	Moderate quality of evidence
		1.6.2. Ultrasound is not recommended in adolescents.	Moderate quality of evidence
		1.6.3. Anti-müllerian (AMH) levels are not recommended in diagnosis in those within 8 years of menarche	Strong quality of evidence
		1.6.4. Adolescents "at risk" can be identified, where diagnosis is unclear, with follow-up reassessment 8 years postmenarche or age of 18 years.	Moderate quality of evidence

Contd...

Contd...

No.	Question for recommendation	Recommendation	Quality of evidence
1.7.	**What are the diagnostic criteria for diagnosis of PCOS in perimenopausal and postmenopausal women?**	1.7.1. A diagnosis of PCOS could be considered enduring/lifelong.	Moderate quality of evidence
		1.7.2. When there is past diagnosis, or a long-term history of oligo-amenorrhea with hyperandrogenism and/or PCOM, during the earlier reproductive years (age 20–40).	Moderate quality of evidence
		1.7.3. Both clinical and biochemical hyperandrogenism persist in postmenopause in women with PCOS.	Moderate quality of evidence
		1.7.4. One should investigate to rule out androgen-secreting tumors and ovarian hyperthecosis in those presenting with new-onset, severe or worsening hyperandrogenism including hirsutism.	Moderate quality of evidence
1.8.	**What are the screening tests and clinical signs for cardiovascular risk?**	1.8.1. PCOS women are at increased risk of cardiovascular disease and potentially of cardiovascular mortality and therefore regardless of age and BMI, should have a lipid profile (cholesterol, low density lipoprotein cholesterol, high-density lipoprotein cholesterol, and triglyceride level) assessed at diagnosis.	Moderate quality of evidence
		1.8.2. Thereafter, frequency of measurement should be based on the presence of hyperlipidemia and additional risk factors.	Clinical practice point
		1.8.3. All women with PCOS should have blood pressure measured annually and when planning pregnancy or seeking fertility treatment, given the high risk of hypertensive disorders.	Moderate quality of evidence
		1.8.4. Healthcare providers should prioritize preventative strategies to reduce cardiovascular risk.	Moderate quality of evidence

Contd...

Contd...

No.	Question for recommendation	Recommendation	Quality of evidence
1.9.	**What are the screening test and clinical signs of insulin resistance?**	1.9.1. Insulin resistance is common in women with PCOS irrespective of age and BMI, which is manifested as an increased risk of impaired fasting glucose, impaired glucose tolerance and type 2 diabetes mellitus.	Strong quality of evidence
		1.9.2. Glycemic status should be assessed at diagnosis of PCOS in all adults and adolescents and should be reassessed every 1–3 years, based on additional individual risk factors for diabetes.	Strong quality of evidence
		1.9.3. Clinically, one must look for signs of acanthosis nigricans and truncal obesity.	Moderate quality of evidence
		1.9.4. 75 g of OGTT should be done with or without HbA1c.	Moderate quality of evidence
		1.9.5. If the OGTT cannot be performed, fasting plasma glucose and/or glycated hemoglobin (HbA1c) could be considered, though it has a significantly reduced accuracy.	Moderate quality of evidence
		1.9.6. Insulin levels should not be done to assay variability (depending on age, gender, and feeding status) and inaccuracy (absence of validated assay).	Moderate quality of evidence
1.10.	**What is the risk in relatives?**	1.10.1. Healthcare professionals could consider that fathers and brothers of women with PCOS may have an increased prevalence of metabolic syndrome, type 2 diabetes mellitus, and hypertension.	Moderate quality of evidence
		1.10.2. Healthcare professionals, adults, and adolescents with PCOS, and their first-degree relatives should be aware of the increased risk of diabetes and the need for regular glycemic assessment.	Moderate quality of evidence
		1.10.3. The cardiometabolic risk in female first-degree relatives of women with PCOS remains inconclusive.	Clinical practice point

Contd...

Contd...

No.	Question for recommendation	Recommendation	Quality of evidence
2.	**Lean versus Obese Polycystic Ovarian Syndrome**		
2.1.	**What are nutritional and environmental influences throughout the life course and the perpetuation of the transgenerational inheritance of PCOS?**	2.1.1. Nutritional and environmental influences throughout the life course and the perpetuation of the transgenerational inheritance is seen in PCOS.	Low quality of evidence
		2.1.2. Poor quality diet, overnutrition, sedentary behavior, obesity, emotional stress, circadian rhythm disruption, poor gut health, or environmental chemical exposure (both intrauterine and after birth results in altered fetal programming with high risk of PCOS.	Low quality of evidence
		2.1.3 Genetic and epigenetic intrauterine growth programming results in a developmentally programmed thrifty genotype (obesity, premature adrenarche, and pubarche and metabolic syndrome) with activation of thrifty phenotype during childhood and adolescence that results in the development of PCOS in adulthood with increased risk of obesity, type II diabetes, metabolic syndrome, and fatty liver.	Low quality of evidence
		2.1.4. Obesity, IR, compensatory hyperinsulinemia along with chronic low-grade inflammatory state influence the clinical and metabolic parameters of PCOS.	Clinical consensus statement
2.2.	**Why are women with PCOS at increased risk of weight gain and Central Obesity?**	2.2.1. Visceral adiposity in PCOS is associated with increased IR, leading to exacerbation of reproductive and metabolic abnormalities.	Low quality of evidence
		2.2.2. Overeating, decreased physical activity, stress, developmental priming and epigenetics, and deficiency in magnesium, chromium, potassium, and vitamins E and C are responsible for visceral obesity.	Clinical practice point

Contd...

Contd...

No.	Question for recommendation	Recommendation	Quality of evidence
2.3.	**How important is visceral obesity in pathogenesis and clinical manifestation of PCOS?**	2.3.1. Androgens influence visceral adiposity, which decreases adiponectin, induces leptin resistance and lipogenesis with high number of cortisol receptor in visceral adipose tissue that can result in increased cortisol response with increased activity of 5-α-reductase.	Moderate quality of evidence
		2.3.2. Visceral obesity results in metabolic and reproductive disturbances thus increases the manifestations of PCOS (insulin resistance, decreased insulin sensitivity, and increased dyslipidemia, ↑menstrual/ovulatory disturbances, ↑hyperandrogenism, ↓SHBG, ↓fertility and ↑pregnancy complications.	High-quality of evidence
		2.3.3. Visceral obesity results in neurohormonal activation and chronic inflammation which in turn increases the risk of metabolic syndrome.	Moderate quality of evidence
		2.3.4. It is recommended that screening women with PCOS for obesity by BMI and for visceral obesity by measuring waist circumference as it can influence the phenotype.	Low quality of evidence
2.4.	**Is lean PCOS also obese and why?**	2.4.1. Lean PCOS also has visceral adiposity with less muscle mass (Sarcopenic).	Moderate quality of evidence
		2.4.2. Sarcopenia adds to altered insulin function and manifestations of hyperandrogenism and metabolic disturbances in women with PCOS.	Low-quality of evidence
		2.4.3. Lean PCOS should be counseled regarding vigilance for progression to metabolic syndrome.	Clinical practice point
		2.4.4. Moderate physical activity and strength training exercise are recommended in women with lean PCOS to counter the metabolic issues associated with sarcopenia and PCOS.	Moderate quality evidence

Contd...

Contd...

No.	Question for recommendation	Recommendation	Quality of evidence
2.5.	**Why are South Asians more prone to insulin resistance?**	2.5.1. South Asian Phenotype carries more fat with same BMI and have a higher risk of developing insulin resistance than other ethnic populations owing to evolution and genetic predisposition.	Moderate quality of evidence
		2.5.2. South Asians have more total and visceral fat with less lean mass, skeletal muscle, bone mineral density, and lower β-cell population compared to ethnic groups, which increase insulin resistance and further risk of metabolic syndrome.	Moderate quality of evidence
2.6.	**What are the similarities and differences between lean and obese PCOS?**	2.6.1. Similar prevalence of acanthosis nigricans, menstrual dysfunction, hirsutism, and endometrial hyperplasia in both lean and overweight.	Moderate quality of evidence
		2.6.2. Hormonal profiles were also similar with respect to LH:FSH ratio, serum LH, progesterone and testosterone levels.	Moderate quality of evidence
		2.6.3. Both have insulin resistance and hyperinsulinemia with a prevalence of 83.3% and 93.1% in lean and overweight respectively.	High quality of evidence
		2.6.4. No difference between lean and obese on pelvic ultrasound features, viz., volume, AFC, and stroma.	Moderate quality of evidence
		2.6.5. Hormonal and metabolic imbalances are more frequently encountered in obese PCOS women.	High quality of evidence
		2.6.6. Android obesity, high triglyceride, and cholesterol levels are the only parameters that vary between obese and lean, being higher in obese PCOS.	High quality of evidence

Contd...

Contd...

No.	Question for recommendation	Recommendation	Quality of evidence
2.7.	**Is obesity associated with greater reproductive dysfunction?**	2.7.1. Obesity is associated with menstrual dysfunction and can lead to precocious menarche (<9 years), irregular cycles, and oligo-/amenorrhea.	High quality of evidence
		2.7.2. Obesity is also associated with sexual dysfunction—difficulty of performance and impairment of desire, arousal, and orgasm.	Low quality of evidence
		2.7.3. Incidence of infertility is three times higher in obese PCOS.	High quality of evidence
		2.7.4. Obesity influences treatment of infertility with poor response to fertility drugs, requirement for higher dose of gonadotropins, altered endometrial function, lower success rates with ART due to altered ovarian responsiveness and oocyte quality and decreased oocytes retrieved and a higher incidence of cancellation of cycle.	High quality of evidence
		2.7.5. Implantation, clinical pregnancy rate (CPR), and live birthrate (LBR) progressively worsen with increasing BMI with a higher incidence of miscarriage rate.	High quality of evidence
		2.7.6. BMI >29 kg/m^2 is associated with reduced success of ongoing pregnancy and a 4% lower pregnancy rate per/kg/m^2 BMI increase.	Moderate quality of evidence
		2.7.7. Obesity in PCOS results in increased time to conception.	Low quality of evidence
2.8.	**What is the treatment for lean and obese PCOS?**	2.8.1. Assessment with an interdisciplinary team taking into consideration BMI and other chronic conditions is essential.	Moderate quality of evidence
		2.8.2. Lifestyle changes are beneficial for weight loss, maintaining weight and building muscle mass in both obese and lean PCOS.	High quality of evidence
		2.8.3. Therapeutic interventions such as combined oral contraceptives, antiandrogens, and insulin sensitizers are helpful in treating symptoms related to anovulation, hyperandrogenemia, and insulin resistance.	High quality of evidence

Contd...

Contd...

No.	***Question for recommendation***	***Recommendation***	***Quality of evidence***
		2.8.4. Metformin, an insulin sensitizer, was more successful in restoring menstruation (55%) and ovulation (45%) in lean women with PCOS compared with their obese counterparts.	Moderate quality of evidence
		2.8.5. 3 g/day of myoinositol appeared to have a positive effect on lean women with PCOS, which led to reductions in luteinizing hormone, androgen levels, "high-sensitivity C-reactive protein" and facilitated insulin tolerance.	Very low quality of evidence
		2.8.6. Suppression of ovarian androgen production using oral contraceptive preparations, Androgen receptor blockers [cyproterone acetate, flutamide, spironolactone, and 5-α-reductase inhibitors (finasteride)] and cosmetic treatment (hair removal by electrolysis or laser therapy is useful to reduce hair growth.	High quality of evidence
		2.8.7. Mild and moderate cases of acne may respond to topical preparations such as benzylperoxide and/or clindamycin or retinoid creams, whereas severe cases may need additional oral treatment with a tetracycline group of antibiotics and in some cases oral isotretinoin.	Low quality of evidence
		2.8.8. Progesterone therapy protects the endometrium in both lean and obese PCOS.	Moderate quality of evidence
		2.8.9. There is no evidence of a beneficial impact of short-term weight loss on LBR after IVF treatment or pregnancy outcome.	Low quality of evidence
		2.8.10. Surgical techniques such as unilateral or bilateral laparoscopic ovarian drilling was found to be associated with comparable rates of successful pregnancies between lean and obese PCOS.	Moderate quality of evidence

Contd...

Contd...

No.	*Question for recommendation*	*Recommendation*	*Quality of evidence*
		2.8.11. Bariatric surgery may be an option in women with a BMI of >35 kg/m^2 and the presence of comorbidities. Bariatric surgery does not improve the clinical live birthrate in women with PCOS and high BMI.	Moderate quality of evidence
		2.8.12. In obese women, lifestyle modification previous to IVF does not enhance embryo utilization or cumulative live birth rate. The duration it takes to lose weight may not be beneficial in combating the problems of declining ovarian reserve.	Moderate quality of evidence
		2.8.13. Lean women with PCOS exhibited a significantly higher rate of fertilization compared with their overweight counterparts (BMI ≥25 kg/m^2).	Low quality of evidence
3.	**Screening and Management of Mental Health in Polycystic Ovary Syndrome**		
3.1.	**What is the prevalence and severity of reduced quality of life?**	3.1.1. PCOS has adverse impact on quality of life in adults.	Moderate quality of evidence
		3.1.2. All PCOS women should be asked about their perception of PCOS symptoms, in particular, impact on quality of life, and what are the key concerns and priorities for the management of their symptoms.	Clinical practice point
3.2.	**What is the prevalence and severity of anxiety and depression?**	3.2.1. The clinician should be aware of the high prevalence of anxiety symptoms and disorders and moderate to severe depressive symptoms and depression in adults and adolescents with PCOS.	Strong quality of evidence
		3.2.2. All clinicians should screen both adolescents and adult women for depression using regionally validated screening tools.	Strong quality of evidence
		3.2.3. If moderate or severe depressive or anxiety symptoms are detected, the patient should be further assessed, counseled and, if necessary, referred to a psychologist or psychiatrist for appropriate treatment.	Strong quality of evidence

Contd...

Contd...

No.	***Question for recommendation***	***Recommendation***	***Quality of evidence***
		3.2.4. The screening for anxiety and depression should ideally be done at the time of diagnosis of PCOS with repeat screening if necessary. No fixed interval is recommended and reassessment should be based on clinical judgment, risk factors, comorbidities and life events.	Clinical practice point
		3.2.5. Screening for mental health disorders comprises assessment of risk factors, symptoms, and risk of deliberate self-harm and suicidal intent.	Clinical practice point
3.3.	**What is the prevalence and severity of body image distress?**	3.3.1. Clinicians should be aware that features of PCOS can have a negative impact on body image.	Strong quality of evidence
3.4.	**What is the prevalence and severity of psychosexual dysfunction?**	3.4.1. Though exact prevalence not known, PCOS women present with variable psychosexual dysfunction that influence fertility, mood disorders, and require medications.	Low quality of evidence
		3.4.2. Clinicians should discuss psychosexual function with couples which may be related to their psychological condition.	Low quality of evidence
3.5.	**What is the prevalence and severity of eating disorders?**	3.5.1. Eating disorders including anorexia nervosa; bulimia nervosa and binge-eating disorder should be enquired in all PCOS patients irrespective of the weight as these are common and may influence management.	Low quality of evidence
		3.5.2. If eating disorders are suspected, further assessment with appropriate management should be offered.	Clinical practice point

Contd...

Contd...

No.	Question for recommendation	Recommendation	Quality of evidence
3.6.	**What are the different psychological and therapeutic options that can be offered for the management and support of depression and/or anxiety or disordered eating?**	3.6.1. Clinicians should provide tailored information, education and information resources that is high-quality, culturally appropriate and inclusive to all with PCOS in a timely, respectful and empathic manner.	Moderate quality of evidence
		3.6.2. A multidisciplinary approach for counseling and screening is necessary involving trained clinicians who could apply evidence-based knowledge for counseling.	Low quality of evidence
		3.6.3. Appropriate time should be given during the consultation, which helps shared decision-making for further management options.	Low quality of evidence
		3.6.4. Women with disordered eating, body image distress, low self-esteem, or psychosexual dysfunction should be offered Psychological therapy (cognitive behavioral therapy) as first-line management besides additional antianxiolytics and antidepressant medications if deemed necessary in adults where anxiety and depression are clearly documented and those with suicidal tendency.	Low quality of evidence
		3.6.5. Overlooking management of anxiety and depression may impact adherence to PCOS treatment to improve overall QoL.	Clinical practice point
4.	**Lifestyle Management**		
4.1.	**Diet and Nutrition**		
4.1.1.	**Are lifestyle interventions effective for improving anthropometric, metabolic, reproductive, fertility, quality of life, and emotional well-being outcomes?**	4.1.1.1. Lifestyle intervention (exercise alone or multicomponent diet combined with exercise and behavioral strategies) should be recommended for all women with PCOS, to improve anthropometric, metabolic, reproductive, fertility, quality of life, and emotional well-being outcomes.	Strong quality of evidence
		4.1.1.2. Every individual with PCOS should undergo a thorough assessment of their lifestyle, including diet, exercise, sleep patterns, emotional well-being, stress levels (both work-related and personal), and current quality of life.	Clinical consensus

Contd...

Contd...

No.	Question for recommendation	Recommendation	Quality of evidence
		4.1.1.3 To facilitate this, a standardized and user-friendly questionnaire should be developed, enabling patients to provide information to healthcare professionals for effective interpretation.	Clinical practice point
		4.1.1.4. Interventions should be delivered by a multidisciplinary team that includes a dietitian, physiotherapist, psychologist, besides clinicians ensuring a holistic approach to care.	Clinical practice point
		4.1.1.5. Healthcare providers should create a personalized lifestyle prescription tailored to the specific needs and circumstances of individuals.	Clinical practice point
4.1.2.	**What are the dietary interventions that are effective for improving anthropometric, metabolic, reproductive, fertility, quality of life, and emotional well-being outcomes?**	4.1.2.1. A personalized energy deficit should be prescribed for women requiring weight loss, depending on individual energy requirements, bodyweight, and physical activity levels.	Clinical practice point
		4.1.2.2. Women with PCOS should be advised to follow a hypocaloric diet rich in whole grains, lean proteins, healthy fats, and low glycemic index foods. Reducing the intake of refined carbohydrates and sugars is crucial.	Clinical practice point
		4.1.2.3. Including anti-inflammatory foods and traditional Indian spices like turmeric and fenugreek may offer additional benefits.	Clinical practice point
		4.1.2.4. Including nuts and oil seeds as sources of good quality fats and protein will compensate for the reduction in carbohydrates.	Clinical practice point
4.1.3.	**How would you counsel the women with PCOS regarding diet for maintaining the weight?**	4.1.3.1. The concept of "diet" needs to be changed to a "healthy eating pattern" as the word "diet" is perceived to be something very restrictive and generates a sense of deprivation among people and a perception that they cannot follow it for long.	Clinical practice point

Contd...

Contd...

No.	Question for recommendation	Recommendation	Quality of evidence
		4.1.3.2. Dietary counseling for women with PCOS should emphasize the importance of a balanced diet, portion control for creating negative calorie balance, and regular meal timings. Counseling should focus on the benefits of low glycemic index foods, high fiber intake, and regular physical activity. Behavioral strategies like mindful eating and keeping a food diary should also be encouraged.	Clinical practice point
		4.1.3.3. Counseling should emphasize on making "healthy eating" as a pattern for the entire family as these dietary changes are good for the entire family's metabolic health.	Clinical practice point
		4.1.3.4. Dietitians with optimal knowledge of eating habits should be involved in counseling.	Clinical practice point
		4.1.3.5. Women with PCOS should be counseled for a lifelong focus on diet for weight loss and prevention of further weight gain.	Clinical practice point
		4.1.3.6. For those who are not overweight, they should be counseled to focus on a healthy lifestyle which includes diet and exercise to prevent excess weight gain.	Clinical practice point
4.1.4.	**Barriers to weight loss?**	4.1.4.1. Weight loss for women with PCOS should be approached as a collaborative effort between the patient and a multidisciplinary team of healthcare professionals (HCPs), including clinicians, dietitians, exercise physiologists, and mental health specialists.	Clinical practice point
		4.1.4.2. A coordinated and one-stop solution that integrates medical, nutritional, psychological, and exercise support is crucial for effective management.	Clinical practice point
		4.1.4.3. Patient-centric approach, tailored to the individual's unique needs, is more effective than generalized guidelines.	Clinical practice point

Contd...

Contd...

No.	Question for recommendation	Recommendation	Quality of evidence
		4.1.4.4. Delivering scientific facts and knowledge in an empathetic manner to improve motivation.	Clinical practice point
		4.1.4.5. Support groups help to create awareness among patients and family members alike.	Clinical practice point
4.2.	**Exercise and Yoga**		
4.2.1.	**What are the components one needs to look at when recommending exercise and yoga to women with PCOS?**	4.2.1.1. An initial assessment for comorbidities, current physical activity, eating habits and disorders, and quality of life is necessary. Subsequently, anthropometric and cardiovascular risk assessment (waist circumference, BMI, and blood pressure) and exercise tolerance (cardiorespiratory fitness, muscle strength, exercise capacity, and physical limitations) need to be evaluated using validated self-administration questionnaires.	Clinical practice point
		4.2.1.2. Assessment and reassessment of cardiorespiratory fitness and muscular strength, power, and endurance, may be effective strategies to increase exercise self-efficacy given their responsiveness to exercise interventions, particularly among those who are physically inactive or exercise-naïve.	Clinical practice point
		4.2.1.3. Yoga therapy can be a preferred choice to incorporate into a patient's daily routine to optimize other lifestyle interventions and treatments.	Clinical practice point
		4.2.1.4. There is a lack of evidence supporting any one type and intensity of exercise to improve anthropometric, metabolic, hormonal, and reproductive or psychological outcomes.	Moderate quality of evidence

Contd...

Contd...

No.	Question for recommendation	Recommendation	Quality of evidence
4.2.2.	**Are exercise interventions effective for improving anthropometric, metabolic, reproductive, fertility, quality of life, and emotional well-being outcomes?**	4.2.2.1. The available evidence, including mechanistic studies, shows that exercise interventions can improve a variety of cardiometabolic health outcomes in PCOS, including insulin sensitivity, central obesity, and cardiorespiratory fitness.	Low quality of evidence
		4.2.2.2. Exercise intervention can improve quality of life and emotional well-being.	Low quality of evidence
		4.2.2.3. Exercise has been shown to improve central adiposity and reduce cardiovascular disease risk.	Clinical practice point
		4.2.2.4. Yoga therapy may significantly decrease menstrual irregularity, clinical hyperandrogenism, fasting blood glucose, fasting insulin, and homeostatic model assessment-insulin resistance value.	Low quality of evidence
4.2.3.	**Is exercise also important in Lean PCOS?**	4.2.3.1. Physical activity is important for lean PCOS women with a focus on a healthy lifestyle and prevent weight gain.	Clinical practice point
		4.2.3.2. Lean PCOS have low muscle mass thus, strength training exercises and low-impact yoga practice would be beneficial.	Clinical practice point
		4.2.3.3. Yoga and meditation have an effective role in managing day-to-day stress levels and psychological health.	Clinical practice point
4.2.4.	**What exercise would you advise for obese and lean PCOS?**	4.2.4.1. For both obese and lean PCOS, a balanced exercise regimen is beneficial, although the regimen may need individualization.	Clinical practice point
		4.2.4.2. Any physical activity consistent with population guidelines will have health benefits and within this, healthcare professionals should advise sustainable physical activity based on individual preferences and goals.	Low quality of evidence

Contd...

Contd...

No.	***Question for recommendation***	***Recommendation***	***Quality of evidence***
		4.2.4.3. All adults should undertake physical activity as doing some physical activity is better than none. Adults should limit the amount of time spent being sedentary (e.g., sitting and screen time) as replacing sedentary time with physical activity of any intensity (including light intensity) provides health benefits.	Clinical practice point
		4.2.4.4. For the prevention of weight gain and maintenance of health, adults (18–64 years) should aim for a minimum of 150–300 minutes of moderate-intensity or 75–150 minutes of vigorous-intensity aerobic activity per week or an equivalent combination of both spread throughout the week, plus muscle-strengthening activities (e.g., resistance/flexibility) on two nonconsecutive days per week.	Low quality of evidence
		4.2.4.5. For the promotion of greater health benefits, including modest weight loss and prevention of weight regain, adults (18–64 years) should aim for a minimum of 250 minutes of moderate-intensity or 150 minutes of vigorous-intensity aerobic activity per week or an equivalent combination of both spread throughout the week, plus muscle-strengthening activities (e.g., resistance/flexibility) on two nonconsecutive days per week.	Low quality of evidence
		4.2.4.6. Adolescents should aim for at least 60 minutes of moderate-to-vigorous—intensity physical activity per day, including activities that strengthen muscle and bone, at least three times per week.	Low quality of evidence
		4.2.4.7. For patient who prefers yoga therapy can practice 10 minutes of meditation and 20 minutes of dynamic asana postures under a trained yoga therapist five times a week.	Low quality of evidence

Contd...

Contd...

No.	Question for recommendation	Recommendation	Quality of evidence
4.2.5.	**How would you counsel women with PCOS regarding Exercise and Yoga for maintaining weight?**	4.2.5.1. Counseling should involve motivational interviewing, questions directed at barriers in weight loss, and identifying which barriers are crossed with ease which are moderate and which are extremely difficult.	Clinical practice point
		4.2.5.2. Patients have to come out with a commitment to start with minor changes, to begin with, and a time-bound plan to attempt to cross major barriers.	Clinical practice point
		4.2.5.3. Identify support systems at home/work/social media.	Clinical practice point
		4.2.5.4. Referral to trained allied healthcare professionals may help in optimizing physical activity.	Clinical practice point
		4.2.5.5. Journaling changes	Clinical practice point
		4.2.5.6. Reporting to mentor	Clinical practice point
4.2.6.	**What are the barriers to weight loss?**	4.2.6.1. Barriers to weight loss are similar to barriers to lifestyle changes in general.	Clinical practice point
		4.2.6.2. The difficulty in achieving and sustaining weight loss in PCOS can be attributed to a variety of physiological, psychological, and socioeconomic factors.	Low quality of evidence
		4.2.6.3. Key barriers to weight loss can be at individual-level (e.g., time and financial pressure, psychological comorbidities, and lack of motivation for maintaining a healthy lifestyle), treatment-related (e.g., high cost and long duration of treatment, and no relief of symptoms), system-level (e.g., lack of professional support and empathy, and unavailability of allied health professionals), and environmental barriers (e.g., lack of social support and exercise environment), insulin resistance, and hormonal imbalance can make weight loss difficult.	Low quality of evidence
		4.2.6.4. Regular follow-ups are necessary at weekly intervals, for 3 months. Then at monthly intervals for 6 months and then every 3 months thereafter.	Clinical practice point
		4.2.6.5. At 3 months intervals, it is important to evaluate them on patient-reported outcomes such as quality of life and levels of sleep quality and anxiety.	Clinical practice point

Contd...

Contd...

No.	*Question for recommendation*	*Recommendation*	*Quality of evidence*
4.3.	**Behavioral Strategies for Polycystic Ovary Syndrome**		
4.3.1.	**What is the effect of PCOS on the psychological well-being and personality of women?**	4.3.1.1. Psychological well-being is severely impacted in women with PCOS causing significant morbidity.	Clinical practice point
		4.3.1.2. All PCOS women should be questioned to assess traits such as impulsivity, reward-seeking behavior, self-control, and conscientiousness.	Clinical practice point
		4.3.1.3. Those women showing signs of anxiety or depression should be offered lifestyle interventions, psychotherapy, and if needed medical treatment.	Strong recommendation but low quality of evidence
4.3.2.	**Can behavior modification interventions aid in the management of PCOS?**	4.3.2.1. The clinician should be aware of the various behavior modification interventions that can be offered to women with PCOS.	Clinical Practice point
		4.3.2.2. Behavior modification interventions help to optimize psychological and emotional well-being of women suffering from PCOS.	Clinical Practice point
		4.3.2.3. Behavioral strategies such as goal setting, self-monitoring, problem-solving assertiveness training, reinforcing changes, and relapse prevention to optimize weight management, healthy lifestyle, and emotional well-being in women with PCOS.	Moderate quality of evidence
		4.3.2.4. They must be counseled to improve adherence to and sustainability of other measures taken for the management of PCOS like diet, exercise, and pharmacotherapy.	Clinical Practice point
4.3.3.	**What is the utility of mindfulness programs in managing PCOS?**	4.3.3.1. Integration of meditation with conventional treatment modalities of management in PCOS women may improve QoL.	Clinical practice point

Contd...

Contd...

No.	Question for recommendation	Recommendation	Quality of evidence
		4.3.3.2. Mindfulness interventions may improve psychosocial well-being and QoL in women with PCOS and therefore can be used as an adjunct to conventional treatment in women with PCOS.	Clinical practice point
		4.3.3.3. Meditation and mindfulness-based healthy lifestyle may improve psychological and metabolic parameters in PCOS women.	Very low quality of evidence
		4.3.3.4. Depression Anxiety Stress Scales (DASS-21) scale should be used to monitor the psychological distress in patients.	Low quality of evidence
4.3.4.	**What is the role of cognitive behavioral therapy in the management of PCOS?**	4.3.4.1. Cognitive behavioral therapy (CBT) has well-characterized benefits in, improving the patient's quality of life.	Low quality of evidence
		4.3.4.2. Cognitive behavioral therapy helps in alleviating diseases associated with depression, anxiety, and obesity that can help in improving quality of life in women with PCOS.	Low quality of evidence
		4.3.4.3. Clinicians should screen PCOS patients for psychological distress and refer those positive to a psychiatrist for cognitive behavioral therapy.	Clinical practice points
4.3.5.	**What is the consensus regarding use of traditional, complementary, and integrative medicine (TCIM) in PCOS?**	4.3.5.1. TCIM approaches may play an important role in the ongoing treatment regimen to help to provide culturally sensitive patient-centred care.	Clinical practice point
		4.3.5.2. Yoga helps to improve overall health of women with PCOS.	Clinical practice point
		4.3.5.3. One on one or group yoga sessions specifically tailored for PCOS should be encouraged and organized.	Clinical practice point
		4.3.5.4. TCIM can be used for symptoms that are not managed by current medical approaches.	Clinical practice point

Contd...

Contd...

No.	Question for recommendation	Recommendation	Quality of evidence
5.	**Management of Nonfertility Signs and Symptoms**		
5.1.	**Cosmetic Measures**		
5.1.1.	**What is the treatment for acne?**	5.1.1.1. For mild to moderate acne—IGA Grade 2-3: Combination of topical benzoyl peroxide either a face wash or cream/gel, along with topical retinoids like adapalene or tretinoin.	High quality of evidence
		5.1.1.2. For moderate to severe acne—IGA Grade 3-4 without hyperandrogenism: Oral antibiotics like doxycycline/minocycline with the topical benzoyl peroxide and retinoids application. For moderate to severe acne—i.e., IGA Grade 3-4 with diagnosed hyperandrogenism: Hormonal therapies with the newer generation oral contraceptive pills. If no response or suboptimal response add spironolactone.	Moderate quality of evidence
		5.1.1.3. For severe nodulocystic or resistant acne: Oral isotretinoin with or without hormonal therapy. With topical agents like benzoyl peroxide/azelaic acid	High quality of evidence
		5.1.1.4. All the grades can be supplemented by azelaic acid, salicylic acid gels/serums along with cosmetic procedures for better results.	Clinical practice point
5.1.2.	**What is the treatment for Hirsutism?**	5.1.2.1. For mild cases of hirsutism and patient-important hirsutism pharmacological therapy with OCPs alone as the first line of therapy.	Moderate quality of evidence
		5.1.2.2. For mild cases of hirsutism in patients who do not wish to conceive/have completed their family—Antiandrogens alone.	Low quality of evidence

Contd...

Contd...

No.	Question for recommendation	Recommendation	Quality of evidence
		5.1.2.3. For moderate to severe cases of hirsutism—OCPs with antiandrogens.	Moderate quality of evidence
		5.1.2.4. For cases of patient-important hirsutism/mild cases where there is no response even after 6 months of monotherapy with OCPs add an antiandrogen alone. Continue the treatment for at least 6–9 months to label it as nonresponsive.	Low quality of evidence
		5.1.2.5. For hirsutism in females with high risk for venous thromboembolism—use a OCP with low dose ethinylestradiol and a low-risk progestin.	Moderate quality of evidence
		5.1.2.6. For all cases of hirsutism—laser hair reduction for dark hairs and electrolysis for gray hair is preferable to the temporary methods of hair removal alone.	Low quality of evidence
		5.1.2.7. One needs to offer holistic treatment including lifestyle changes to all patients of hirsutism irrespective of the severity of the hirsutism. Treatments should be designed taking into consideration the patient's needs and desires.	Clinical practice point
5.1.3.	**What is the treatment for acanthosis nigricans?**	5.1.3.1. In cases of acanthosis nigricans with obesity—weight reduction, metformin, along with treatment of underlying PCOS.	Low quality of evidence
		5.1.3.2. In cases of acanthosis nigricans without obesity treatment should be directed to underlying PCOS.	Low quality of evidence
		5.1.3.3. Topical treatment can be added to all cases. Tretinoin 0.05–0.1% cream/gel application or calcipotriol 0.05%.	Low quality of evidence
		5.1.3.4. Cosmetic treatments are to be suggested as per the severity of the condition and the patient's requirements.	Clinical practice point

Contd...

Contd...

No.	Question for recommendation	Recommendation	Quality of evidence
5.1.4.	**What is the treatment for female pattern hair loss?**	5.1.4.1. Topical minoxidil 5% application.	High quality of evidence
		5.1.4.2. Treatment of hyperandrogenemia with Spironolactone and oral combined contraceptive pills of third- and fourth-generation results in improvement.	Moderate quality of evidence
		5.1.4.3. Low-level of light therapy and PRP.	Low quality of evidence
5.1.5.	**How effective are cosmetic procedures?**	5.1.5.1. Cosmetic procedures like lasers, chemical peels, PRP are additive and do work synergistically with medical therapy and are effective in reducing dermatological manifestations.	Moderate quality of evidence
5.2.	**Pharmacotherapy**		
5.2.1.	**What is the role of combined oral contraceptives (COCP)?**	5.2.1.1. The combined oral contraceptive pill (COCP) is recommended in reproductive-age women with PCOS for the management of hirsutism and/or irregular menstrual cycles.	Moderate quality of evidence
		5.2.1.2. The COCP could be used in adolescents at risk or with a clear diagnosis of PCOS for management of hirsutism and/or irregular menstrual cycles.	Moderate quality of evidence
		5.2.1.3. Low dose of ethinylestradiol (<30 µg) in the COCP is preferred for treating hirsutism.	Moderate quality of evidence
		5.2.1.4. The 35 µg ethinylestradiol with cyproterone acetate should be used only as second-line therapy over other COCPs, as it is associated with adverse effects, including venous thromboembolic risks.	Moderate quality of evidence
		5.2.1.5. Progestin-only oral contraceptives may be considered for endometrial protection, though the evidence in women with PCOS is limited.	Low quality of evidence

Contd...

Contd...

No.	*Question for recommendation*	*Recommendation*	*Quality of evidence*
5.2.2.	**Which is the most effective and safest COCP available and how long should they be continued?**	5.2.2.1. Estrogen-containing COCP is effective and recommended in the treatment of inflammatory acne in females.	High quality of evidence
		5.2.2.2. Both ethinylestradiol/drospirenone and ethinylestradiol/cyproterone acetate combinations improve hyperandrogenic parameters significantly without affecting the insulin resistance adversely in Indian women with PCOS.	High quality of evidence
		5.2.2.3. Progestin-only oral contraceptives may be considered for endometrial protection.	Moderate quality of evidence
		5.2.2.4. Use of lowest effective dose of 20–30 µg of ethinylestradiol or equivalent is effective and safe.	Clinical practice points
		5.2.2.5. COCPs could be given for 3–6 months for cycle regulation.	Clinical practice points
		5.2.2.6. COCPs could be given for 6 months for a reduction in hirsutism and acne.	Clinical practice points
		5.2.2.7. OCPs need to be stopped in the presence of any side effects or if abnormal glucose tolerance or dyslipidemia is detected.	Low quality of evidence
		5.2.2.8. After initial evaluation with all contraindications ruled out COCPs can be given for longer periods and regular follow-up advised.	Clinical practice points
5.2.3.	**What precautions one needs to take when prescribing COCP in adolescents and adults?**	5.2.3.1. While prescribing COCPs to women with PCOS, the relative and absolute contraindications and side effects of COCPs need to be considered.	Clinical practice point
		5.2.3.2. COCPs chosen should not worsen the metabolic profile of the woman with PCOS.	Clinical practice point

Contd...

Contd...

No.	*Question for recommendation*	*Recommendation*	*Quality of evidence*
5.2.4.	**What is the role of Insulin sensitizers (metformin and myoinositols) and should all women with PCOS be given insulin sensitizers?**	5.2.4.1. Metformin offers greater benefits in high metabolic risk groups including those with diabetes risk factors, and impaired glucose tolerance.	Clinical practice point
		5.2.4.2. Metformin alone should be considered in adults with PCOS and a BMI ≥25 kg/m² for anthropometric and metabolic outcomes including insulin resistance, glucose, and lipid profiles.	Very low quality of evidence
		5.2.4.3. Could be given to adolescents with BMI ≥25 kg/m² for the management of weight and metabolic outcomes if LSM is not effective.	Very low quality of evidence
		5.2.4.4. Where COCP is contraindicated, not accepted or not tolerated, metformin may be considered for irregular menstrual cycles.	Clinical practice point
		5.2.4.5. Myoinositol, part of the vitamin B complex, could be considered for women with PCOS, noting limited harm, and potential for improvement in metabolic measures.	Very low quality of evidence
		5.2.4.6. Metformin + myoinositol combination treatment in obese patients with PCOS has demonstrated better improvement in hormonal and metabolic parameters compared to metformin or myoinositol alone.	Clinical practice point
		5.2.5.7. Metformin is to be considered over inositol in hirsutism and central obesity.	Very low quality of evidence
		5.2.5.8. First-line therapy which should be recommended to all women with PCOS is lifestyle intervention (behavior, diet, and physical activity).	Very low quality of evidence
		5.2.4.9. Insulin sensitizers should be given in women with BMI >25 and/or those who have glucose intolerance.	Very low quality of evidence
		5.2.4.10. Insulin sensitizers which include metformin and inositols are indicated when lifestyle intervention is not effective.	Clinical practice point

Contd...

Contd...

No.	*Question for recommendation*	*Recommendation*	*Quality of evidence*
5.2.5.	**How long to continue Insulin sensitizers in adolescents and adults?**	5.2.5.1. Insulin sensitizers should be continued in the presence of impaired glucose tolerance and type 2 diabetes mellitus.	High quality of evidence
		5.2.5.2. Could be used for more than 6 months in woman without impaired glucose tolerance or type 2 diabetes with regular follow ups, for better and sustained weight loss.	Clinical practice point
		5.2.5.3. Insulin sensitizers could be given as an adjunct to lifestyle intervention for a duration of 6 months.	Clinical practice point
5.2.6.	**Is combination therapy of COCP and metformin more beneficial?**	5.2.6.1. COCP therapy has benefits for management of hyperandrogenism and menstrual regulation and metformin has beneficial effects on metabolic profile.	Clinical practice point
		5.2.6.2. Metformin and COCP combination could work better in adults with PCOS with a BMI > 30 kg/m^2, diabetes risk factors, impaired glucose tolerance or high-risk ethnic groups.	Clinical practice point
		5.2.6.3. Combination of COCPs and metformin could be recommended in adults and adolescents with obesity/metabolic complications when lifestyle modification (LSM) and COCP is not effective.	Clinical practice point
5.2.7.	**What is the role of antiandrogens and which group of women benefit from antiandrogen therapy?**	5.2.7.1. Antiandrogens are effective in treating hirsutism.	Very low quality of evidence
		5.2.7.2. Antiandrogens with COCPs could be tried for managing alopecia.	Low quality of evidence
		5.2.7.3. Women on antiandrogen therapy should avoid pregnancy.	Clinical practice point
		5.2.7.4. Antiandrogens could be given to manage hirsutism, where 6 months of COCP and/or cosmetic therapy is not effective.	Very low quality of evidence
		5.2.7.5. Antiandrogens could be given to treat hirsutism in women in whom COCP are either contraindicated or not tolerated.	Clinical practice point

Contd...

Contd...

No.	*Question for recommendation*	*Recommendation*	*Quality of evidence*
5.2.8.	**Should antiandrogens be used in combination with other drugs to be more effective?**	5.2.8.1. Antiandrogens can be used to treat hirsutism with effective contraception if there is suboptimal response with 6 months of treatment with COCP and or cosmetic therapy or where there is a contraindication for use of COCP or when COCPs are poorly tolerated.	Very low quality of evidence
		5.2.8.2. Antiandrogens with COCPs could be tried for managing alopecia and to correct menstrual irregularity.	Very low quality of evidence
		5.2.8.3. In case there is pregnancy when antiandrogens are used there is a risk of incomplete development of external genital structures of male fetuses.	Clinical practice point
5.3.	**Role of Antiobesity Drugs in Adolescents and Adult Women with PCOS**		
5.3.1.	**What are antiobesity drugs used for weight reduction and which of them are available in India?**	5.3.1.1. Orlistat, phentermine/topiramate, naltrexone/bupropion, glucagon-like peptide-1 (GLP-1) receptor agonists-liraglutide, and semaglutide are approved for nonsyndromic obesity. Tirzepatide and incretins are currently being investigated in different phases of clinical trials.	Low quality of evidence
		5.3.1.2. Orlistat, liraglutide, semaglutide, and tirzepatide are the drugs available in India apart from the ayurvedic drugs used for weight loss.	Clinical practice point
		5.3.1.3. Antiobesity medications like glucagon-like peptide-1 (GLP-1) receptor (liraglutide and semaglutide), and orlistat, could be used in addition to active lifestyle interventions, for the management of obese PCOS.	Very low quality of evidence
		5.3.1.4. Combining medications with complementary mechanisms of action could be a management strategy in those who are unable to maintain weight loss or have further weight loss after reaching a weight loss plateau.	Low quality of evidence

Contd...

Contd...

No.	***Question for recommendation***	***Recommendation***	***Quality of evidence***
5.3.2.	**Are antiobesity medications effective as per the evidence from large clinical trials, systematic reviews and meta-analyses?**	5.3.2.1. The currently available antiobesity medications are effective in the management of obesity in women and result in at least 5% weight loss at the end of 1 year of treatment.	Moderate quality of evidence
5.3.3.	**What are the advantages and disadvantages of the antiobesity agents currently available?**	5.3.3.1. Use of orlistat is associated with oily rectal leakage, abdominal distress, abdominal pain, flatulence with discharge, fecal urgency, steatorrhea, fecal incontinence, and increased defecation.	Very low quality of evidence
		5.3.3.2. The use of liraglutide is associated with increased heart rate, hypoglycemia, constipation, diarrhea, nausea, vomiting, and headache.	Low quality of evidence
		5.3.3.3. The use of semaglutide is associated with nausea, vomiting, diarrhea, abdominal pain, constipation, and headache.	Very low quality of evidence
		5.3.3.4. Use of phentermine/topiramate is associated with elevation in heart rate, mood and sleep disorders, cognitive impairment, metabolic acidosis, paresthesia, and dry mouth.	Very low quality of evidence
5.3.4.	**What are the contraindications for using antiobesity medicine?**	5.3.4.1. Antiobesity drugs can be used as long as there is no contraindication for their use and do not result in significant side-effects.	Low quality of evidence
5.3.5.	**How long should the antiobesity drugs be administered?**	5.3.5.1. The length of time one takes antiobesity drugs depends on weight loss and whether one experiences any serious side effects.	Clinical practice point

Contd...

Contd...

No.	Question for recommendation	Recommendation	Quality of evidence
5.4.	**Role of Bariatric Surgery in PCOS**		
5.4.1.	**Is bariatric/metabolic surgery effective for the management of hormonal and clinical PCOS features and weight?**	5.4.1.1. Bariatric surgery in the forms of LSG and RYGB is effective in normalizing metabolic parameters such as triglycerides, fasting glucose, fasting insulin, HOMA-IR, HbA1C but also improving SHBG, lowering testosterone and free androgen index.	Low quality of evidence
		5.4.1.2. The effect on AMH levels is conflicting.	Very low quality of evidence
5.4.2.	**What are the indications for bariatric Surgery in adolescents and adults?**	5.4.2.1. For adolescents, bariatric surgery should be considered after evaluation by a multidisciplinary team in the presence of overweight (BMI is at or above the 85th percentile and below the 97th percentile) or severe obesity (BMI above the 97th percentile) and those who have previously participated in lifestyle interventions with unsuccessful outcomes. • Class II obesity—BMI >120% of the 95th percentile with comorbidity • Class III obesity—BMI >140% of the 95th percentile	Low quality of evidence
		5.4.2.2. In adults bariatric surgery should be considered depending on the BMI and presence or absence of comorbidities. • Obese—BMI >35 kg/m2 regardless of comorbidities • BMI >30 kg/m2 with type 2 diabetes mellitus • Class I obesity—BMI of 30–34.9 kg/m2 who do not achieve substantial or durable weight loss or comorbidity improvement using nonsurgical methods	Low quality of evidence
		5.4.2.3. Bariatric surgery is not recommended for PCOS per se.	Clinical practice point

Contd...

Contd...

No.	***Question for recommendation***	***Recommendation***	***Quality of evidence***
5.4.3.	**What are the maternal and fetal complications of bariatric surgery?**	5.4.3.1. Bariatric surgery may result in nutritional deficiencies, anemia, altered maternal glucose metabolism and small for gestational age children, which may then result in adverse outcomes both in the mother and neonate. Women are therefore counseled to use effective contraception immediately before surgery or after surgery to delay conception for 1–1.5 years to prevent maternal and neonatal complications.	Low quality of evidence
		5.4.3.2. Bariatric surgeries may significantly reduce the occurrence of obesity-related complications during pregnancy like GDM, PIH, PE, and CSs.	Moderate quality of evidence
		5.4.3.3. Maternal and perinatal outcomes differ according to type of bariatric surgery and serious surgical complications are more common with gastric bypass than gastric banding. Therefore the choice of bariatric surgery should take into account the impact of surgery on future pregnancy.	Low quality of evidence
5.4.4.	**Can bariatric surgery influence the fertility and pregnancy outcome?**	5.4.4.1. Bariatric surgery has a positive impact on the pregnancy with increased chance of spontaneous conception or a better success rate after ART.	Low quality of evidence
		5.4.4.2. Female sexual dysfunction (FSD) is resolved after bariatric surgery as assessed by female sexual function index (FSFI).	Low quality of evidence
		5.4.4.3. Little is known about the effect of bariatric surgery on breastfeeding, so it should not be restricted after bariatric surgery.	Very low quality of evidence

Contd...

Contd...

No.	***Question for recommendation***	***Recommendation***	***Quality of evidence***
5.5.	**Common Sleep Disorders in Polycystic Ovary Syndrome**		
5.5.1.	**What are the PCOS effects on sleep?**	5.5.1.1. PCOS has an adverse effect on the sleep quality and thereby daytime functioning.	Moderate to high quality of evidence
		5.5.1.2. Sleep health evaluation to diagnose underlying sleep disorders especially OSA is essential.	Moderate to high quality of evidence
5.5.2.	**What is the pathophysiology of sleep disorders?**	5.5.2.1. Anatomic factors (such as micrognathia, large tongue as in acromegaly, hypothyroidism), large neck circumference, increased bony structures and soft tissues around the neck as seen in obesity increase the risk of obstructive sleep apnea (OSA). These features should be looked for in individual patients.	Moderate to high quality of evidence
		5.5.2.2. Upper airway collapsibility and pharyngeal narrowing is worsened by upper airway dilator hypo responsiveness, high loop gain, low arousal threshold and reduced ventilatory drive during sleep.	Low to moderate quality of evidence
5.5.3.	**What is the prevalence, evaluation and treatment options for snoring and OSA in PCOS?**	5.5.3.1. OSA forms the most common sleep disorder described in patients with PCOS.	High quality of evidence
		5.5.3.2. When there is a high clinical probability for OSA as assessed by symptoms and clinical evaluation including questionnaires, diagnosis should always be confirmed by sleep studies.	High quality of evidence
		5.5.3.3. Treatment options include lifestyle changes, continuous positive airway pressure therapy when severe or symptomatic and if that fails, consideration of a mandibular advancement device as in non-PCOS.	Moderate quality of evidence

Contd...

Contd...

No.	Question for recommendation	Recommendation	Quality of evidence
5.5.4.	**How to evaluate and treat Insomnia in PCOS?**	5.5.4.1. Chronic insomnia in PCOS needs to be teased out further to see whether it is an independent association or part of the mood disturbances that is very common in PCOS.	High quality of evidence
		5.5.4.2. Insomnia should be effectively treated to improve quality of life.	High quality of evidence
5.5.5.	**What is the management of Restless legs (RLS, Willis–Ekbom Disease) in PCOS?**	5.5.5.1. PCOS patients should be specifically asked for restless legs when sleep health is being evaluated.	Low quality of evidence
6. Screening and Management for Infertility till Intrauterine Insemination			
6.1.	**What are the preconception risk factors associated with poor or negative fertility outcomes?**	6.1.1. The preconception risk factors associated with poor or negative fertility outcomes are: i. Maternal age >35 years ii. Obesity with BMI >30 kg/m^2 iii. *Number of cycles:* >3 previous cycles of IUI iv. *Type of infertility:* Primary infertility v. Duration of infertility of >4.8 years	Low quality of evidence
		6.1.2. In PCOS women planning for pregnancy it is important to evaluate weight, blood pressure, lipid profile, lifestyle including addictions, nutrition, exercise, and sleep.	Low quality of evidence
		6.1.3. One should optimize the reproductive outcome by healthy lifestyle, prevention of excess weight gain, and optimizing preconception risk factors, mental, emotional, and sexual health.	Clinical practice point

Contd...

Contd...

No.	Question for recommendation	Recommendation	Quality of evidence
		6.1.4. Chronic conditions such as diabetes, high blood pressure, anxiety, depression, and other mental health conditions should be optimally managed and women should be counseled regarding the risk of adverse pregnancy outcomes.	Clinical practice point
6.2.	**Is it necessary to confirm that patient is anovulatory before starting any treatment?**	6.2.1. Since OI cycles are associated with better results than natural cycles irrespective of ovulatory status of the woman, confirmation of anovulation before starting treatment is not necessary.	Low quality of evidence
6.3.	**What test would you do before inducing ovulation?**	6.3.1. To diagnose PCOS one must exclude other disorders with following tests.	Low quality of evidence
		6.3.2. In women with PCOS and infertility due to anovulation alone with normal semen analysis, the risks, benefits, costs, and timing and techniques of tubal patency testing in relation to the cost and complexity of the treatment should be considered on an individual basis, depending on personal history and population prevalence, prior to starting ovulation induction with timed intercourse or intrauterine insemination.	Moderate quality of evidence
		6.3.3. Free androgen index by testing total testosterone and SHBG may be necessary in the absence of clinical hyperandrogenemia.	Moderate quality of evidence
		6.3.4. Baseline ultrasound to rule out any other pelvic abnormality and for estimating the AFC.	Low quality of evidence
		6.3.5. Testing for impaired glucose tolerance, lipid profile, and metabolic disorders is essential.	Moderate quality of evidence

Contd...

Contd...

No.	***Question for recommendation***	***Recommendation***	***Quality of evidence***
6.4.	**Which oral ovulogens will you use and why?**	6.4.1. Letrozole should be the first-line pharmacological treatment for ovulation induction in infertile anovulatory women with PCOS, with no other infertility factors.	High quality of evidence
		6.4.2. The use of letrozole is still off-label in many countries, where it is not allowed, clinicians should use other ovulation induction agents.	Clinical practice point
		6.4.3. Clomiphene citrate could be used as a second-line pharmacological treatment for ovulation induction.	Moderate quality of evidence
		6.4.4. Metformin could be used alone, in women with PCOS with anovulatory infertility and, to improve clinical pregnancy and live birthrates, after informing women that there are more effective ovulation agents.	High quality of evidence
		6.4.5. Clomiphene citrate combined with metformin could be used rather than clomiphene citrate or metformin alone in women with PCOS with anovulatory infertility to improve ovulation and clinical pregnancy rates.	Moderate quality of evidence
		6.4.6. Current evidence demonstrates no difference in fetal abnormality rates between letrozole and/or clomiphene citrate ovulation induction or natural conception.	Clinical practice point
6.5.	**How will you manage resistance to oral ovulogens?**	6.5.1. Lifestyle modification with diet and exercise to keep BMI between 19 and 30 kg/m^2 is recommended. But, one must take into consideration the age of the patient as with increasing age the chance of conception decreases.	High quality of evidence
		6.5.2. Addition of metformin may be beneficial when combined with clomiphene citrate to induce ovulation in addition to correcting hyperinsulinemia.	Moderate quality of evidence

Contd...

Contd...

No.	Question for recommendation	Recommendation	Quality of evidence
		6.5.3. Glucocorticoids may be given in resistant cases.	Low quality of evidence
		6.5.4. Alternative options for OI in case of resistance include: a. Extended therapy of letrozole and clomiphene citrate b. Change the oral ovulogen c. Combination of Letrozole and clomiphene citrate	Low quality of evidence
		6.5.5. Gonadotropins could be second-line pharmacological therapy for women with PCOS who are anovulatory with oral ovulogens. Gonadotrophins could be used alone or in combination with letrozole and clomiphene citrate.	Moderate quality of evidence
		6.5.6. Laparoscopic ovarian drilling (LOD) could be second-line therapy for women with PCOS who are anovulatory and infertile, with clomiphene citrate resistance.	Moderate quality of evidence
		6.5.7. IVF could be offered in women with PCOS and anovulatory infertility, if first- or second-line ovulation induction therapies have failed.	Moderate quality of evidence
7. Role of ART in PCOS: Increasing Efficiency and Reducing Complications			
7.1.	**What are the indications for ART in women with PCOS?**	7.1.1. In PCOS women with anovulatory infertility, IVF/ICSI is recommended when first- or second-line ovulation induction treatment have failed or in the presence of absolute indication like tubal factor, male factor, severe endometriosis, low ovarian reserve or when PGT is required to prevent aneuploidy and genetically inherited disease.	Low quality of evidence
7.2.	**What is the COS protocol of choice?**	7.2.1. The antagonist protocol is recommended as it allows the use of GnRH agonist trigger with the freezing of all embryos generated, if required, without compromising the cumulative live birth rate, to reduce the risk of ovarian hyperstimulation syndrome (OHSS).	High quality of evidence

Contd...

Contd...

No.	*Question for recommendation*	*Recommendation*	*Quality of evidence*
		7.2.2. There is insufficient evidence to recommend a particular type of gonadotropin preparation. Either urinary or recombinant follicle stimulating hormone (FSH) or human menopausal hormone (hMG) could be used in women with PCOS undergoing controlled ovarian hyperstimulation for IVF/ICSI.	Very low quality of evidence
7.3.	**How will you prevent OHSS in women with PCOS?**	7.3.1. It is recommended to proceed with antagonist protocol to reduce the risk of moderate and severe OHSS in high responders or high-serum estradiol levels.	High quality of evidence
		7.3.2. As a first line strategy, it is recommended to use GnRH agonist as trigger for oocyte maturation to reduce the risk of OHSS.	High quality of evidence
		7.3.3. It is recommended for freeze all strategy and subsequent frozen embryo transfer to reduce the risk for early and late onset OHSS.	High quality of evidence
		7.3.4. It is recommended to individualize the dose of gonadotropins based on the ovarian reserve tests.	Moderate quality of evidence
		7.3.5. The risk of OHSS is increased when there are more than 17–19 mature follicles and elevated serum estradiol levels on the day of the trigger (greater than 3,500–5,000 pg/mL), as well as when more than 15–18 oocytes are retrieved.	High quality of evidence
		7.3.6. In patients at risk for moderate-to-severe OHSS, it is recommended to start cabergoline on the day of trigger or soon thereafter and continue for several days. Usually, it is administered in the dose of 0.5 mg once daily for 8 days.	High quality of evidence
		7.3.7. It is not recommended to use low dose of hCG only as trigger to reduce the risk of OHSS.	Low quality of evidence

Contd...

Contd...

No.	Question for recommendation	Recommendation	Quality of evidence
		7.3.8. It is not recommended to administer letrozole to reduce the risk of moderate or severe OHSS as an intervention.	Moderate quality of evidence
		7.3.9. Volume expanders such as albumin, hydroxyethyl starch, and mannitol are not recommended as a preventive strategy for moderate or severe PCOS.	Low quality of evidence
		7.3.10. There is no recommendation to use Aspirin, mifepristone, myoinositol, D-chiro-inositol, or glucocorticoids to reduce OHSS risk.	Low quality of evidence
		7.3.11. The administration of a GnRH antagonist in the luteal phase is proposed to accelerate luteolysis, reduces ovarian VEGF secretion, and promotes the regression of OHSS symptoms. However, the evidence does not support the use of a GnRH antagonist alone postretrieval to reduce the risk of moderate to severe OHSS.	Low quality of evidence
		7.3.12. Coasting is not recommended as a primary strategy to reduce the risk of OHSS. However, it can be considered alongside other strategies, such as cabergoline and the freeze-all strategy, if more effective options are unavailable.	Low quality of evidence
7.4.	**How will you manage OHSS?**	7.4.1. Outpatient management is considered in patients with mild or moderate OHSS and selected cases of severe OHSS.	Very low quality of evidence
		7.4.2. Women undergoing outpatient management of OHSS should be counseled regarding fluid intake and output monitoring and they should be provided with contact details to access advice.	Very low quality of evidence
		7.4.3. Nonsteroidal anti-inflammatory agents should be avoided, as they may compromise renal function.	Very low quality of evidence

Contd...

Contd...

No.	Question for recommendation	Recommendation	Quality of evidence
		7.4.4. Women with severe OHSS being managed on an outpatient basis should receive thromboprophylaxis with LMWH. The duration of treatment should be individualized, based on risk factors and whether conception occurs or not.	Very low quality of evidence
		7.4.5. Paracentesis of ascitic fluid may be carried out on an outpatient basis by the abdominal or transvaginal route under ultrasound guidance.	Very low quality of evidence
		7.4.6. There is insufficient evidence to support the use of GnRH antagonists or dopamine agonists in treating established cases of OHSS.	Very low quality of evidence
7.5.	**Is in vitro maturation (IVM) of oocytes treatment of choice in women with PCOS?**	7.5.1. IVM should be considered only when there is sufficient expertise, as an option in women with prior severe OHSS and with increased risk in present stimulation, acknowledging the lower cumulative livebirth rate.	Moderate quality of evidence
		7.5.2. Evidence suggests that IVM/ICSI is less effective than standard IVF/ICSI in terms of clinical pregnancy and livebirth rate per patient.	Clinical practice points
7.6.	**Should metformin be used in all patients undergoing ART?**	7.6.1. It is not recommended to give metformin for the sole purpose of reducing OHSS in PCOS women in GnRH antagonist cycles. However, it can be considered to reduce the risk of OHSS in women undergoing GnRH agonist protocol.	Moderate quality of evidence
		7.6.2. It can be considered in women with hirsutism, insulin resistance and central obesity.	Very low quality of evidence

Contd...

Contd...

No.	*Question for recommendation*	*Recommendation*	*Quality of evidence*
7.7.	**How important is lifestyle modification in patients who need ART? What is the evidence?**	7.7.1. Lifestyle intervention (exercise alone or multicomponent diet combined with exercise and behavioral strategies) should be recommended for all women with PCOS, for improving metabolic health including central adiposity and lipid profile.	High quality of evidence
		7.7.2. Healthy lifestyle behavior includes healthy eating and/or physical activity and is recommended in all PCOS women to optimize general health, quality of life, body composition, and weight management.	High quality of evidence
		7.7.3. *Exercise intervention:* It is recommended to encourage these women to undertake physical activity. They should aim for a minimum of 150–300 minutes of moderate intensity activity or 75–150 minutes of vigorous intensity aerobic activity per week or combination of both spread throughout the week along with muscle strengthening activities on two nonconsecutive days per week.	High quality of evidence
		7.7.4. As per 2023, PCOS guidelines, there is no evidence to support one type of diet composition over the other. The diet composition should be consistent with the population guidelines and should advice healthy eating tailored to individual goals and preferences.	Clinical practice point
7.8.	**How to prevent complications in ART?**	7.8.1. To prevent the risk of developing OHSS, it is preferred to plan antagonist protocol with agonist trigger and freeze all strategy.	High quality of evidence
		7.8.2. If fresh embryo transfer is planned, one should opt for single embryo transfer to prevent occurrence of multiple pregnancy.	High quality of evidence

Contd...

Contd...

No.	Question for recommendation	Recommendation	Quality of evidence
7.9.	**What is the role of freeze all in PCOS women undergoing ART?**	7.9.1. It is recommended to consider freeze all strategy and plan for frozen embryo transfer in a subsequent cycle in patients at risk for OHSS, with past history of OHSS with gonadotropin therapy and in those requiring PGT to rule out aneuploidy or single gene disorders.	High quality of evidence
7.10.	**How will you prepare the endometrium for FET?**	7.10.1. Natural or stimulated cycle FET is preferred over HRT as the relaxin and other substances from the corpus luteum prevents the pregnancy complications like preeclampsia, diabetes mellitus, preterm labor, and intrauterine growth restriction.	High quality of evidence
8. Pregnancy Outcome in Women with Polycystic Ovarian Syndrome			
8.1.	**Are women with PCOS at increased risk of adverse pregnancy outcomes and why?**	8.1.1. Women with PCOS have an increased risk of adverse pregnancy outcomes, which should be identified during antenatal care.	Moderate quality of evidence
		8.1.2. Polycystic ovarian syndrome is associated with infertility, hyperandrogenemia, hyperinsulinemia with insulin resistance (IR), obesity, dyslipidemia, and chronic inflammation and these factors increase the risk of adverse pregnancy outcomes.	High quality of evidence
		8.1.3. Assisted reproductive technology in women with PCOS does not confer an additional risk of miscarriage, preterm birth, impaired fetal growth and cesarean section, over that observed in women without PCOS.	Low quality of evidence
		8.1.4. Polycystic ovarian syndrome women with pregnancy need increased surveillance during pregnancy and delivery to identify the risk factors of adverse pregnancy outcomes and prevent complications.	Clinical practice point

Contd...

Contd...

No.	*Question for recommendation*	*Recommendation*	*Quality of evidence*
8.2.	**What risks have been associated with pregnancy in women with PCOS and how do you prevent them?**	8.2.1. Pregnant women with PCOS have an increased risk of gestational weight gain, miscarriage, gestational diabetes, hypertensive disease during pregnancy, preeclampsia, intrauterine growth restriction, small for gestational age babies and low birth weight, preterm delivery, and cesarean section.	Moderate quality of evidence
		8.2.2. Early lifestyle intervention should be offered to pregnant women with PCOS, given the risk of higher baseline weight, impaired glucose tolerance, dyslipidemia, excess gestational weight gain, and pregnancy complications.	Moderate quality of evidence
		8.2.3. Preconceptional counseling, care, and preparation for pregnancy will prevent complications.	Clinical practice point
		8.2.4. Blood pressure measurement and OGTT should be performed when planning for a pregnancy or seeking fertility treatment.	Clinical practice point
		8.2.5. If OGTT is not performed in the preconception period, it should be done at the first antenatal visit and repeated at 24–28 weeks' gestation.	Clinical practice point
		8.2.6. Proper antenatal screening is helpful to diagnose and manage the adverse effects of pregnancy as early as possible.	Clinical practice point
8.3.	**Should Insulin sensitizers be given prophylactically to prevent complications of pregnancy?**	8.3.1. Healthcare professionals should be aware that metformin in pregnant women with PCOS has not been shown to prevent: • Gestational diabetes • Late miscarriage (12 weeks +1 day to 21 weeks +6 days gestational age) • Hypertension in pregnancy • Preeclampsia • Macrosomia or birthweight ≥4,000 g	

Contd...

Contd...

No.	Question for recommendation	Recommendation	Quality of evidence
		8.3.2. Metformin could be considered in some circumstances (e.g., risk for preterm birth), to reduce preterm delivery and limit excess gestational weight gain, in pregnant women with PCOS.	Moderate quality of evidence
		8.3.3. Women should be counseled that the consequences of metformin exposure on long-term offspring health remain unclear and there is a suggestion of increased childhood weight, although causality is not certain.	Clinical practice point
		8.3.4. Clinicians should know about transplacental and endometrial transmission of insulin sensitizers and when to start and when to stop during pregnancy.	Low quality of evidence
		8.3.5. Clinicians should discuss with the patients about the side effects of insulin sensitizers.	Clinical practice point
8.4.	**How obesity adds to the complications in pregnancy?**	8.4.1. Obesity in PCOS is primarily associated with increased risk of HDP, GDM, and operative deliveries when compared to women with PCOS and BMI <30 kg/m^2.	Low quality of evidence
		8.4.2. Diet and lifestyle modifications to optimize weight-control before pregnancy and adjusting treatment for comorbidities is of importance.	Clinical practice point
9. Long-term Health Implications and Comorbidities of PCOS			
9.1.	**What is the prevalence of long-term health implications and comorbidities?**	9.1.1. Clinicians should be aware that women with PCOS have an increased risk of HTN, T2D, cardiovascular disease, nonfatal cerebrovascular disease events, and adverse lipid profiles compared to those without PCOS.	High quality of evidence

Contd...

Contd...

No.	***Question for recommendation***	***Recommendation***	***Quality of evidence***
		9.1.2. Women diagnosed with PCOS should be counseled about the possible long-term health implications and comorbidities.	Clinical practice point
		9.1.3. Clinicians should screen women with PCOS at diagnosis for impaired glucose tolerance, hypertension and hyperlipidemia and schedule regular follow-ups based on initial results and risk factors.	Clinical practice point
9.2.	**Impaired glucose tolerance and type 2 diabetes—prevention, diagnosis, and management?**	9.2.1. Clinicians should inform women with PCOS about their increased risk of impaired fasting glucose, IGT and T2D regardless of age and BMI.	High quality of evidence
		9.2.2. Glycemic status should be evaluated at diagnosis of PCOS and rechecked every 1–3 years, based on individual risk factors for T2D.	Moderate quality of evidence
		9.2.3. Clinicians should recommend the 75 g OGTT to all women with PCOS, regardless of BMI. If an OGTT cannot be performed, FPG or HbA1C may be done, although their accuracy would be significantly lower. FPG is more sensitive than HbA1C.	Low quality of evidence
		9.2.4. An OGTT should be advised to all women with PCOS and without preexisting diabetes when planning a pregnancy or seeking fertility treatment. If preconception OGTT is not performed, it should be performed at the first antenatal visit. All women with PCOS should be tested at 24–28 weeks of gestation.	Low quality of evidence
		9.2.5. The key intervention to prevent progression to T2D, especially in those who are overweight and obese, are lifestyle modifications comprising dietary interventions and physical activity.	Clinical practice point
		9.2.6. The use of insulin-sensitizing agents, along with lifestyle interventions may improve their metabolic profile.	Clinical practice point

Contd...

Contd...

No.	Question for recommendation	Recommendation	Quality of evidence
9.3.	**How to prevent, diagnose and manage cardiovascular risks?**	9.3.1. Women with PCOS should be informed about increased CVD risk and the potential of cardiovascular mortality and should be screened for its risk factors.	Moderate quality of evidence
		9.3.2. At diagnosis, women with PCOS should have a lipid profile (cholesterol, LDL-C, HDL-C and triglyceride level). Test frequency should be determined by the presence or absence of hyperlipidemia and additional risk factors.	Moderate quality of evidence
		9.3.3. Women with PCOS should have BP and weight measured at least once a year.	Low quality of evidence
		9.3.4. Clinicians should inform women with PCOS that lifestyle interventions is the first-line approach in modifying the risk of CVD. Adherence to a healthy diet, regular exercise, and weight reduction are the key components of prevention.	Clinical practice point
		9.3.5. Metformin, glucagon-like peptide-1 receptor agonists and SGLT-2 inhibitors may reduce CVD risk in insulin-resistant women by improving lipid profile and BMI.	Moderate quality of evidence
		9.3.6. If HTN is diagnosed in women with PCOS it should be controlled to reduce the risk of CVD. The target blood pressure should be <130/80 mm Hg.	Clinical practice point
9.4.	**What are the criteria to diagnose metabolic syndrome?**	9.4.1. Women with PCOS should be informed and screened for MetS and its complications, especially CVD and T2D.	High quality of evidence
		9.4.2. Clinicians should be aware that early diagnosis and treatment of MetS may have a significant impact in reducing mortality and morbidity.	High quality of evidence

Contd...

Contd...

No.	Question for recommendation	Recommendation	Quality of evidence
		9.4.3. For diagnosing metabolic syndrome three out of five criteria of the following should be present (NCEP-ATP III criteria). • Elevated triglycerides: ≥150 mg/dL • Reduced HDL-C: <50 mg/dL • Elevated blood pressure: Systolic ≥130 mm Hg and/or Diastolic ≥85 mm Hg or treated hypertension • Elevated fasting glucose: >100 mg/dL • *Elevated waist circumference:* Central/South American, Chinese, Japanese, South Asian: ≥80 cm Mediterranean, Middle East, Sub-Saharan African: ≥80 cm Europid (includes Canada, Europe, and the United States): ≥88 cm	High quality of evidence
9.5.	**Does the incidence of gynecological malignancies (endometrium, ovaries, and breast) increase in PCOS?**	9.5.1. Clinicians should be aware that premenopausal women with PCOS have a higher risk of developing atypical hyperplasia and endometrial cancer.	High quality of evidence
		9.5.2. Inform women with PCOS of their higher risk for atypical hyperplasia and endometrial cancer. However, since the overall risk of developing endometrial cancer is low, routine screening is not advised.	Clinical practice point
		9.5.3. Long-standing untreated amenorrhea, obesity, type 2 diabetes and persistent thickened endometrium are risk factors for endometrial hyperplasia and endometrial cancer in women with PCOS.	Clinical practice point

Contd...

Contd...

No.	*Question for recommendation*	*Recommendation*	*Quality of evidence*
		9.5.4. Clinicians should be aware that the association of PCOS with ovarian cancer is undetermined.	Clinical practice point
		9.5.5. Clinicians should be aware that the association of PCOS with breast cancer is low.	Moderate quality of evidence
		9.5.6. Clinicians should be aware that the association of PCOS with cervical, fallopian tube and vulvar cancer is undetermined.	Clinical practice point
9.6.	**How to prevent cancer risk in women with PCOS?**	9.6.1. Women with PCOS should be informed about preventive measures, including weight management, menstrual cycle regulation, and regular progesterone therapy to induce withdrawal bleeding at least every 3 months.	Clinical practice point
		9.6.2. When excessive endometrial thickness is detected, a biopsy with histological analysis and a withdrawal bleed should be considered.	Clinical practice point
		9.6.3. Progesterone should always be part of menopausal hormone therapy (MHT) in women with an intact uterus for endometrial protection, except in low dose vaginal estrogen therapy.	Clinical practice point
9.7.	**How do you manage endometrial cancer conservatively?**	9.7.1. Women with PCOS suffering from atypical hyperplasia or grade 1 endometrioid endometrial cancer without myometrial invasion should be counseled that fertility-sparing treatment is not the standard of care. Only those who strongly desire to preserve fertility should pursue this option.	Low quality of evidence
		9.7.2. Patients who are candidates for fertility-preserving treatment must be referred to specialized centers or experienced gyne-oncologists using well-defined protocols.	Clinical practice point

Contd...

Contd...

No.	*Question for recommendation*	*Recommendation*	*Quality of evidence*
9.8.	**Is there an increased risk of inflammation in PCOS?**	9.8.1. Clinicians should be aware that low-grade chronic inflammation overlaps with comorbidities like CVD, dyslipidemia, obesity, and reproductive abnormalities in women with PCOS.	Moderate quality of evidence
		9.8.2. Clinicians should be aware that various inflammatory markers are implicated in the pathophysiology, and considered as biomarkers of PCOS.	Low quality of evidence
9.9.	**What is the prevalence, diagnosis and management of NAFLD and NASH in women with PCOS?**	9.9.1. Clinicians should be highly vigilant and initiate, implement and adjust screening practices to reflect the incidence of NAFLD in PCOS women of all ages and BMI categories.	Moderate quality of evidence
		9.9.2. A gastroenterologist/hepatologist should be involved in the care of women diagnosed with elevated liver enzymes or hepatic steatosis on imaging.	Clinical practice point
9.10.	**How will you prevent the occurrence of late sequelae in PCOS?**	9.10.1. Clinicians should recommend lifestyle changes, including diet, exercise, and weight loss, along with regular monitoring of glucose and lipid metabolism as the first line of treatment for women with PCOS to improve long-term outcomes. These changes should precede and/or accompany any pharmacological treatment.	Low quality of evidence
		9.10.2. Overweight or obese women should be counseled about the benefits of weight loss which include significantly reduced risk of CVD, T2D, MetS, OSA, EC, and NAFLD. In women with excess weight, a weight loss of 5–10% is advised, aiming for an energy deficit of 30% or 500–750 kcal/day (1,200–1,500 kcal/day).	Clinical practice point

Contd...

Contd...

No.	Question for recommendation	Recommendation	Quality of evidence
		9.10.3. Clinicians should be aware that NAFLD is often reversible in its early stages, so early detection is crucial to prevent further liver damage and significantly improve the quality of life.	Clinical practice point
		9.10.4. Bariatric surgery may be considered for morbidly obese women with PCOS, particularly those with a BMI of 40 kg/m^2 or more, or 35 kg/m^2 or more with a high-risk obesity-related condition if standard weight loss strategies have not been successful.	Moderate quality of evidence
10. Patient's Education, Counseling, and Support Groups in Polycystic Ovary Syndrome			
10.1.	What are the characteristics of available models of care implemented in PCOS clinics or services?	10.1.1. Healthcare systems should implement a multidisciplinary approach that includes specialists such as endocrinologists, gynecologists, dietitians, psychologists, dermatologists, and other relevant professionals to tackle PCOS's complex nature.	Strong quality of evidence
		10.1.2. Models should integrate psychological support and social interventions alongside medical treatments.	Moderate quality of evidence
		10.1.3. Adolescent-specific models of care (MoCs) that focus on education, lifestyle interventions, and individualized medical care should be initiated.	Moderate quality of evidence
		10.1.4. Care models should also be developed in the government healthcare system including primary health care which should include healthcare professional training, virtual options and appropriate referral linkages.	Clinical practice point
10.2.	**How can we best support women to navigate the impact of PCOS on family and**	10.2.1. Encourage family involvement in self-management as getting family members involved in PCOS self-management can dramatically improve women's support systems.	Moderate quality of evidence

Contd...

Contd...

No.	*Question for recommendation*	*Recommendation*	*Quality of evidence*
		10.2.2. Implementing the biopsychosocial model which takes into account the biological, psychological, and social aspects of health has the potential to dramatically improve the QoL for women with PCOS.	Moderate quality of evidence
		10.2.3. To decrease the stigma and marginalization, public health educators need to boost societal awareness and education regarding PCOS.	Clinical practice point
		10.2.4. One needs to develop socioculturally sensitive resources and educational materials on PCOS for families of those affected by the condition.	Clinical practice point
10.3.	**What are the key challenges for those with PCOS when interacting with healthcare professionals about PCOS and related features?**	10.3.1. Healthcare providers should be trained in shared decision-making to provide clear, comprehensive information about PCOS, including its symptoms, evidence-based treatment options, lifestyle modifications, counseling, emotional support, and a multidisciplinary approach.	Strong quality of evidence
		10.3.2. Healthcare providers should adhere to standard treatment guidelines and use appropriate resources by healthcare providers.	Clinical practice point
		10.3.3. Delays in diagnosis and treatment should be reduced by streamlining the diagnostic and referral process and enhancing early detection of PCOS in adolescents.	Clinical practice point
		10.3.4. Evidence-based strategies and resources can enhance patient's participation, which includes knowledge, skills, ability, confidence, and willingness to manage their own health and care. (Evidence-based International Guidelines for PCOS 2023).	Clinical practice point
10.4.	**How important are support groups and how do they function?**	10.4.1. Encourage PCOS support groups to provide evidence-based information, peer support, awareness and socioculturally relevant woman-centered care.	Moderate quality of evidence

Contd...

Contd...

No.	Question for recommendation	Recommendation	Quality of evidence
		10.4.2. PCOS support should be encouraged to have long-standing partnerships with healthcare providers, professional agencies, and researchers, making substantial contributions to advocacy and raising awareness.	Clinical practice point
10.5.	**Is a questionnaire necessary before counseling?**	10.5.1. Out of the four databases—PubMed, Medline, Cochrane, and Scopus—we only utilized PubMed and Medline due to our access limitations. After conducting searches with the relevant keywords, we did not find any pertinent articles for this particular question.	
10.6.	**Who should counsel women with PCOS?**	10.6.1. Implementing a multidisciplinary approach for PCOS counseling involves integrating various specialities and expertise to provide a comprehensive and holistic treatment plan.	Moderate quality of evidence
		10.6.2. Psychologists and trained counselors can counsel women with PCOS.	Clinical practice point
10.7.	**Should the counseling be individual or in a group?**	10.7.1. Individual counseling for personalized care is essential as it provides a tailored and personalized approach to care, which will ensure the unique needs and concerns of each person are addressed with specialized attention.	Clinical practice point
		10.7.2. Group counseling for community support and awareness is essential as it fosters a sense of community support and raises awareness, allowing participants to share experiences and insights in a collective environment that promotes mutual understanding and collective growth.	Clinical practice point
10.8.	**Is patient's education an important aspect in managing PCOS?**	10.8.1. Implement comprehensive user-friendly patient's education programs including digital platforms which include multidisciplinary approach for the management of PCOS.	Clinical practice point
		10.8.2. Patient's education should include information regarding access to health care, comorbidities, follow-ups, and support groups.	Clinical practice point

CHAPTER 1

Definition, Prevalence, Diagnosis and Screening of Polycystic Ovarian Syndrome

Chandrika Anand

INTRODUCTION

Polycystic ovarian syndrome (PCOS) is a complex endocrine disorder that affects women of reproductive age and is strongly associated with disturbances in reproductive, metabolic and mental health. The diagnosis of PCOS is based on the Rotterdam Criteria, which requires the presence of two out of three criteria: Menstrual irregularities, clinical or biochemical hyperandrogenemia and polycystic ovarian morphology.[1] The challenges in diagnosis and management are the complexity of the clinical presentation of PCOS in different age groups, the different methodologies of hormone evaluation and emerging treatment options. Often the condition is either underdiagnosed or overdiagnosed. This chapter gives insight into the criteria for diagnosis, conditions that need to be ruled out, clinical evaluation and biochemical investigations. It also includes screening for metabolic dysfunction and cardiovascular disease risk.

1.1. What is the prevalence of PCOS in Adolescents and Adults?

Draft recommendations:

1.1.1. As the Global and Indian prevalence of PCOS has increased, adults and adolescents suspected to have PCOS should have a diagnostic assessment in accordance with the diagnostic algorithm published by international guidelines. *(Moderate quality of evidence)*

1.1.2. A timely diagnosis of PCOS in symptomatic adolescent girls is important for the initiation of appropriate screening and treatment. *(Strong quality of evidence)*

Summary of evidence: Overall prevalence of PCOS varies between 8 and 13%. 30% of all infertility is associated with anovulation, and 85–90% of these are attributed to PCOS. 21–59% of women of reproductive age demonstrate a USG picture of polycystic ovaries and about 30–50% have clinical or biochemical signs of Anovulation and androgen excess.

A meta-analysis by Bharali et al. included 30 studies, mostly from South India and found a pooled prevalence of 11.34% according to the Rotterdam criteria.[2] The global prevalence of PCOS was 9.2% based on a meta-analysis done by Salari et al.[3] It included 35 studies with 12,365,646 subjects and the mean age ranged from 10–45 years.[3] In a systematic review and meta-analysis of 12 studies that included 4,473 participants, the prevalence of PCOS in adolescents was 17.74%.[4] In the adolescent the incidence is higher if the mother has PCOS. Low birthweight and rapid postnatal weight gain with precocious adrenarche/pubarche increase the risk for progression to functional ovarian hyperandrogenism and PCOS in the adolescent.

Research gap: Diagnosis of PCOS has been controversial due to significant clinical heterogeneity, ethnic differences, BMI and changes in symptoms, and clinical features across the lifespan.

1.2. Is there an ethnic variation in the prevalence of PCOS?

Draft recommendations:

1.2.1. There is an ethnic variation in the prevalence as well as clinical presentation and metabolic consequences of PCOS. *(Strong quality of evidence)*

Summary of evidence: Relatively mild phenotypes and higher BMI are seen in Caucasians, especially in those women who are from North America and Australia. More severe hirsutism has been reported in Middle Eastern, Hispanic and Mediterranean women. At the same time, Southeast Asians and Indigenous Australians reported an increased incidence of central adiposity, insulin resistance, DM, metabolic risks and acanthosis nigricans. A lower BMI and milder hirsutism are seen in East Asians, whereas Africans have a higher BMI and metabolic features.[5]

Research gap: Due to ethnic differences in prevalence and clinical presentation across the world, guidelines cannot be applied globally. Due to racial and ethnic-specific differences in PCOS, there could be a lot of disparity in the diagnosis and outcomes associated with PCOS. This warrants future studies to understand the dichotomy and fill the voids in the diagnostic parameters of PCOS.

1.3. Criteria for Diagnosis of PCOS—NIH, Rotterdam, AE-PCOS Society, International guidelines on PCOS 2023

Draft recommendations:

1.3.1. In adult women, it is recommended that a diagnosis of PCOS be made using the modified Rotterdam criteria, meeting two of the following three conditions: *(Strong quality of evidence)*

   I. Androgen excess:

      a. *Clinical:* Persistent acne, hirsutism (A modified Ferriman-Gallwey score of ≥4 to ≥8), female pattern hair loss. Hirsutism should be considered as a strong predictor of hyperandrogenism and PCOS in adults. Acne and alopecia could be considered as being weaker predictors of hyperandrogenism.

b. *Biochemical:*
   - Elevated total or free testosterone, or calculated indices of free testosterone [Free androgen Index (FAI), bioavailable testosterone (BioT)].
   - DHEAS and ANSD can be considered

II. Ovulatory dysfunction: Oligo-amenorrhea (cycles >35 days apart or <8 menses a year). If highly suspicious for PCOS, but does not have oligo-amenorrhea, consider serum progesterone or luteinizing hormone (LH) assessment

III. Polycystic ovary morphology (PCOM) on ultrasound using the new criteria: Follicle number per ovary (FNPO) ≥20 in at least one ovary, follicle number per section (FNPS) ≥10 in at least one ovary or ovarian volume (OV) ≥10 mL. If using the transabdominal approach for USG only volume needs to be reported. The number of follicles is best reported only at a transvaginal scan with a transducer frequency ≥8 MHz

Summary of evidence: There have been four sets of consensus criteria for diagnosing PCOS, each differing slightly in their requirements based on clinical, biochemical, and ultrasound findings[6] **(Table 1)**.

There are four distinct PCOS phenotypes identified using the Rotterdam criteria[1]—androgen excess, ovulatory dysfunction and PCOM,[2] androgen excess and ovulatory dysfunction[3] androgen excess and PCOM,[4] and ovulatory dysfunction and PCOM[7] **(Table 2)**.

Clinical practice guidelines from the Endocrine Society (USA), PCOS Australian Alliance (Australia), the RCOG (UK), and the SOGC (Canada) all endorse the modified Rotterdam criteria for PCOS diagnosis.[8]

Clinical hyperandrogenism should be evaluated by a trained provider and be quantified using the modified Ferriman–Gallwey score. Standardized visual scales such as the modified Ferriman Gallwey score (mFG) should be used to assess hirsutism; ≥8 indicates hirsutism.[9] The mFG cut-off scores for defining hirsutism and the severity of hirsutism vary by ethnicity, and in Indian women ≥7 is diagnostic of hirsutism. Internationally, there are no universally accepted visual assessments for evaluating acne. In India "Indian Acne Association" (IAA) criteria are used for assessing the severity of acne. The Ludwig visual score is preferred to evaluate the degree and distribution of alopecia. Currently, data does not support the use of acne and female pattern hair loss as reliable diagnostic markers for PCOS though commonly seen in women with PCOS.

Biochemical hyperandrogenism should be defined by elevated total or free testosterone, as measured by high-quality assays such as liquid chromatography mass spectrometry and extraction/chromatography

TABLE 1: Summary of all the diagnostic consensus for polycystic ovarian syndrome (PCOS).

Diagnostic consensus	***National Institutes of Health (NIH), 1990***	***Rotterdam, 2003***	***AE-PCOS Society, 2006***	***International Guideline 2023 diagnostic algorithm***
Symptomatic characteristics	1. Clinical or Biochemical hyperandrogenism 2. Ovulation disorder (amenorrhea/ oligomenorrhea) in the absence of nonclassical adrenal hyperplasia	1. Androgen excess/ hyperandrogenism 2. Oligo-ovulation or anovulation 3. Polycystic appearance of the ovaries on ultrasonography. Presence of 12 or more follicles measuring 2–9 mm in diameter on day 2 or 3 of MC and/ or increased ovarian volume (>10 mL) in the absence of dominant follicle >10 mm or CL	1. Hirsutism and/or hyperandrogenemia (clinical or biochemical) 2. Oligo-anovulation and/or polycystic ovarian morphology	1. Step 1: Irregular cycles + clinical hyperandrogenism = Diagnosis 2. Step 2: If no clinical hyperandrogenism Test for biochemical hyperandrogenism = Diagnosis 3. Step 3: If only irregular cycles or hyperandrogenism, ultrasound for PCOM, if positive = Diagnosis Diagnostic criteria for USG diagnosis – Follicle number per ovary (FNPO) ≥20 in at least one ovary – Follicle number per section (FNPS) ≥10 in at least one ovary – Ovarian volume (OV) ≥10 mL
Criteria considered	Patient demonstrates both criteria	Considers any two of three criteria.	Both criteria are required	Two criteria are required

TABLE 2: Different phenotypes of polycystic ovarian syndrome (PCOS).

Parameter	*Phenotype A*	*Phenotype B*	*Phenotype C*	*Phenotype D*
PCOS features	HA/OD/PCOM	HA/OD	HA/PCOM	OD/PCOM
Hyperandrogenism (HA)	✓	✓	✓	
Ovulatory dysfunction (OD)	✓	✓		✓
PCOM features	✓		✓	✓

immunoassay. As these assays may not be available and demonstrate poor sensitivity, accuracy and precision, it is best to assay androgen excess by calculating the free androgen index or bioavailable testosterone.[9] One could evaluate androstenedione and DHEAS if total or free testosterone is not elevated.[9] Interpretation of androgen levels should be guided by the reference ranges of the laboratory used. If the woman is on hormonal contraception, the results may be affected due to its effects on sex hormone-binding globulin (SHBG) and altered gonadotrophin-dependent androgen production.[10]

When irregular menstrual cycles are present a diagnosis of PCOS should be considered and assessed according to the PCOS Guidelines. Oligo-amenorrhea (cycles >35 days apart or <8 cycles per year) may be used as a marker for ovulatory dysfunction to diagnose PCOS. Ovulation can be confirmed with the evaluation of serum progesterone (day 21 and if MC is irregular every 7 days thereafter till menstruation occurs) in those women with uncertain menstrual history.

PCOM should be defined as either ≥20 follicles per ovary and/or an ovarian volume of ≥10 cm^3 of either ovary, using newer transvaginal ultrasound technology with a transducer frequency of 8 MHZ or more.

Serum anti-Müllerian hormone (AMH) has been proposed as an alternative marker of PCOM. AMH correlated with AFC and was significantly higher in women with PCOS. Different AMH assays and differences in age or BMI influence the threshold value for AMH, which makes its diagnostic value controversial.[10]

Research gap: As PCOS is associated with reproductive and metabolic dysfunction and long-term sequelae, a timely and appropriate diagnosis is necessary. With the use of 2003 Rotterdam criteria, PCOS was over diagnosed, which increased the prevalence of PCOS. When diagnosed with PCOS these women are associated with significant psychological distress, reduced well-being, depression, and fears about future health and fertility. Therefore, diagnosis of PCOS should not be given hastily. In future, there should be studies that will identify clinical features that are specific to each phenotype.

1.4. What is new in the diagnosis of PCOS—Role of AMH and ultrasound in PCOS?

Draft recommendations:

1.4.1. Serum AMH could be used for defining PCOM in adult women as an alternative to pelvic ultrasound but should not be used as a single test for the diagnosis of PCOS and should not be used in adolescents for diagnosis. *(Moderate quality of evidence)*

1.4.2. AMH level is not necessary for PCOS diagnosis in patients with irregular menstrual cycles and hyperandrogenism. *(Moderate quality of evidence)*

1.4.3. Age, BMI, use of hormonal contraception, menstrual cycle day and method of assay influence AMH levels. *(Clinical practice point)*

1.4.4. Follicle number per ovary (FNPO) of ≥20, follicle number per cross-section (FNPS) of ≥10 and ovarian volume (OV) of ≥10 mL should be considered accurate ultrasound markers for PCOM in adults. Transvaginal ultrasound is more accurate than transabdominal ultrasound. *(Strong quality of evidence)*

1.4.5. There are no definitive criteria to define polycystic ovary morphology (PCOM) on ultrasound in adolescents, hence it is not recommended in adolescents. *(Clinical practice points)*

1.4.6. Either serum AMH or ultrasound may be used to define PCOM; however, both tests should not be performed to limit overdiagnosis. *(Clinical practice points)*

Quality of evidence: Levels of anti-Müllerian hormone (AMH), secreted by granulosa cells of the preantral and small antral ovarian follicles, are significantly higher among those with PCOS compared to those without PCOS.[11] It has been suggested as a potential marker for ovulatory dysfunction in PCOS and could serve as a standalone diagnostic test. The most commonly proposed cutoff to distinguish women with PCOS from healthy individuals is 35 pmol/L (4.9 ng/mL) using the Beckman Coulter enzyme immunoassay (AMH-EIA), which has a specificity of 97% and superior sensitivity (92%) compared to antral follicle count (AFC). In large epidemiological data sets, where transvaginal ultrasound is not feasible, AMH is a useful tool in PCOS case and phenotype identification when combining the measurement with oligo/amenorrhea and hyperandrogenism.[12]

The former threshold of >12 for follicle number for diagnosis of PCOS is no longer valid, it is 19 with a sensitivity of 81% and specificity of 92%.[13] Higher transducer frequencies (≥8 MHz) have improved the detection of antral follicles, leading to elevated threshold levels.[13] For follicle number per ovary (FNPO) there was a sensitivity of 70–94% and specificity of 70–100% as an ultrasound diagnostic criterion to diagnose PCOS. Follicle number per cross-section (FNPS) demonstrated a sensitivity of 21–94% and specificity of 60–100% as an ultrasound diagnostic criterion to diagnose PCOS.[9] For ovarian volume, there was a sensitivity of 21–94% and specificity of 60–100% as an ultrasound criterion to diagnose PCOS.[9]

In normal adolescent physiology, presence of multi-follicular/PCO is a common feature that decreases with cycle regularity and requires strict interpretation of ultrasonography findings of PCO morphology.[9] Therefore, USG is not recommended in adolescents to diagnose PCOS. Due to declining ovarian function at perimenopausal women, diagnostic criteria with a combination of age, log ovarian volume, follicle number, and testosterone can be used to distinguish PCO morphology.[9]

Research gaps: Although serum AMH levels in adolescent and adults with PCOS are significantly higher than those without PCOS in all studies, there is an overlap between the two groups, especially in adolescents. Factors influencing these thresholds include the use of different AMH assays, age or BMI and whether PCOS or PCOM was excluded in the control population. With automated assays, the variability in the levels of AMH has decreased and hence, a new recommendation on the role of AMH assays in diagnosis of PCOS was made in adults only.

Key challenges with the literature in this area included the variable populations (with and without women with PCOS) used to define cut-off values and the use of the 95th percentile cut-offs to define abnormality. Due to inter- and intraobserver variability, there might be a problem in using ultrasound parameters like ovarian volume; maximum number of follicles in a single sonographic plane; peripheral distribution of ovarian follicles; bright ovarian stroma, and total follicle number for diagnosis of PCOS.

1.5. What criteria indicate ovulatory dysfunction in adolescents?

Draft recommendations:

1.5.1 Irregular cycle and ovulatory dysfunction *(Strong quality of evidence)*
   a. 1 to <3 years postmenarche: <21 or >45 days.
   b. 3 years postmenarche to perimenopause: <21 or >35 days or <8 cycles per year.
   c. 1 year postmenarche >90 days for any one cycle.
   d. Primary amenorrhea by age of 15 years or >3 years postthelarche (breast development).

1.5.2. In adolescents, one needs to identify the optimal timing of assessing PCOM which is physiological at that time. *(Clinical practice point)*

1.5.3. For adolescents who have features of PCOS, but do not meet all three diagnostic criteria, an "increased risk" could be considered and reassessment advised at or before full reproductive maturity, 8 years postmenarche. *(Clinical practice point)*

Summary of evidence: Ovulatory dysfunction is a key diagnostic feature of PCOS, marked by irregular menstrual cycles. The average adult menstrual cycle is 28 days, ranging from 24 to 35 days. Physiologically, during the first-year postmenarche, reproductive hormonal levels do not match adult patterns. The cycles can remain irregular until the fifth-year postmenarche. In adolescents, one needs to identify the optimal timing of assessment as PCOM is physiological during early adolescence and is not associated with abnormalities of ovulation and menstrual cycle duration. Metabolic features like Insulin resistance and increased insulin levels may be seen due to high growth hormone levels, hyper-pulsatile GnRH secretion and decreased levels of SHBG. Increased levels of ovarian and adrenal androgen are also physiological. However, all these abnormalities return to normal at the end of normal puberty but remain elevated in PCOS.

Research gap: However, more frequent cycles do not necessarily indicate ovulation, as ovulatory dysfunction can occur with regular cycles. In such situations, ovulation has to be confirmed by doing serum progesterone levels.

1.6. Can the adult criteria for diagnosis of PCOS be used in adolescent?

Draft recommendations:

1.6.1. A persistent observation of oligo-/amenorrhea beyond 2 years of menarche with either clinical or biochemical hyperandrogenism is a diagnostic criterion of PCOS in adolescents. *(Moderate quality of evidence)*

1.6.2. Ultrasound is not recommended in adolescents. *(Moderate quality of evidence)*

1.6.3. Anti-müllerian (AMH) levels are not recommended in diagnosis in those within 8 years of menarche. *(Strong quality of evidence)*

1.6.4. Adolescents "at risk" can be identified, where diagnosis is unclear, with follow-up reassessment 8 years postmenarche or age of 18 years. *(Moderate quality of evidence)*

Summary of evidence: Diagnosis of PCOS in adolescents is necessary as a timely diagnosis of PCOS in those who are symptomatic is important for the initiation of appropriate screening and treatment Validated diagnostic criteria supported by robust clinical and hormonal findings are needed to avoid overdiagnosis and unnecessary treatment in otherwise healthy normal girls without hyperandrogenism. Normal adolescents do have oligomenorrhea, amenorrhea, acne and "multicystic" ovaries which can be mistaken for PCOS.[9] During adolescence, menstrual irregularities are not proof of adult chronic anovulation. Moreover, at puberty, growth is associated with profound metabolic changes and basal metabolic rate slows at the end of linear growth and predisposes to weight gain. Several metabolic features present at puberty return to normal at the end of normal puberty but remain elevated in PCOS.[5] One must also remember that the later the onset of menarche, the longer until the start of regular menses: <11 years: 14% took >5 years; >17 years: 33% took >5 years.

Suggested criteria for diagnosis of PCOS in adolescents is given in **Table 3**.

Research gaps:

Problems in diagnosis of PCOS in adolescence:

1. Using a broader definition may be problematic
   - Several features may be in evolution, or only be transitory during the transition to adulthood.
   - All Rotterdam criteria may be transient during adolescence.
   - AE-PCOS criteria are more apt but need to be modified to be specific.
2. Prematurely assigning a diagnostic label of PCOS to an adolescent may be incorrect, not needed treatments and worsen psychological distress as PCOS is associated with disorders and therapies involving body image.

1.7. What are the diagnostic criteria for diagnosis of PCOS in perimenopausal and postmenopausal women?

Draft recommendations:

1.7.1. A diagnosis of PCOS could be considered enduring/lifelong. *(Moderate quality of evidence)*

TABLE 3: Criteria for diagnosis of polycystic ovarian syndrome (PCOS) in adolescents.

Required	*Optional (Should not be used independently as diagnostic features)*	*Not recommended (These criteria have been associated with PCOS but are not diagnostic)*	*Comments*
Irregular menses/ oligomenorrhea	PCOM	Obesity	Must generally be 2 years postmenarche
Evidence of hyperandrogenism: a. Biochemical b. Clinical (e.g., progressive hirsutism)	Severe cystic acne	Insulin resistance	Must rule out other disorders of hyperandrogenism (e.g., NC-CAH and Cushing syndrome)
		Hyperinsulinemia	
		Biomarkers (e.g., AMH and T/DHT ratio)	
		Acanthosis nigricans	

1.7.2. When there is past diagnosis, or a long-term history of oligo-amenorrhea with hyperandrogenism and/or PCOM, during the earlier reproductive years (age 20–40). *(Moderate quality of evidence)*

1.7.3. Both clinical and biochemical hyperandrogenism persist in postmenopause in women with PCOS. *(Moderate quality of evidence)*

1.7.4. One should investigate to rule out androgen-secreting tumors and ovarian hyperthecosis in those presenting with new-onset, severe or worsening hyperandrogenism including hirsutism. *(Moderate quality of evidence)*

Summary of evidence: PCOS women have a later menopause than controls. With aging, changes occur in all three diagnostic criteria.[9] Menstrual cycles become more regular in PCOS. Ovarian volume and follicle number decrease longitudinally and are more pronounced. Postmenopausal women with PCOS have higher androgen levels (17-hydroxyprogesterone, androstenedione, DHEAS, total testosterone, and FAI) and lower SHBG levels than women without PCOS.[9] Moreover, postmenopausal women with PCOS report more hirsutism than controls.

Research gaps: Evidence on hyperandrogenism and other features of PCOS in postmenopausal women is more inconsistent. More research is needed to provide clarity on postmenopausal PCOS features.

1.8. What are the screening tests and clinical signs for cardiovascular risk?

Draft recommendations:

1.8.1. PCOS women are at increased risk of cardiovascular disease and potentially of cardiovascular mortality and therefore regardless of age and BMI, should have a lipid profile (cholesterol, low density lipoprotein cholesterol, high-density lipoprotein cholesterol, and triglyceride level) assessed at diagnosis. *(Moderate quality of evidence)*

1.8.2. Thereafter, frequency of measurement should be based on the presence of hyperlipidemia and additional risk factors. *(Clinical practice point)*

1.8.3. All women with PCOS should have blood pressure measured annually and when planning pregnancy or seeking fertility treatment, given the high risk of hypertensive disorders. *(Moderate quality of evidence)*

1.8.4. Healthcare providers should prioritize preventative strategies to reduce cardiovascular risk. *(Moderate quality of evidence)*

Quality of evidence: The quality of evidence for an increase in cardiovascular risk in PCOS is low or very low though the overall incidence rate of cardiovascular disease is significantly higher.[14] The healthcare providers need to encompass assessment of weight, BMI, waist circumference, lipid profiles, blood pressure, glucose levels, and lifestyle in women with PCOS. The risk prediction and assessment tools for females with PCOS should be validated.

Research gaps: The high prevalence of cardiometabolic risk factors is well established, including higher weight, impaired glucose tolerance, diabetes, dyslipidemia, and metabolic syndrome in women with PCOS. Most obstetricians and gynecologists are not fully aware of the long-term serious CVD consequences of PCOS. Creating awareness among clinicians is of prime importance in primary prevention of cardiovascular risk.

1.9. What are the screening test and clinical signs of insulin resistance?

Draft recommendations:

1.9.1. Insulin resistance is common in women with PCOS irrespective of age and BMI, which is manifested as an increased risk of impaired fasting glucose, impaired glucose tolerance and type 2 diabetes mellitus. *(Strong quality of evidence)*

1.9.2. Glycemic status should be assessed at diagnosis of PCOS in all adults and adolescents and should be reassessed every 1–3 years, based on additional individual risk factors for diabetes. *(Strong quality of evidence)*

1.9.3. Clinically, one must look for signs of acanthosis nigricans and truncal obesity. *(Moderate quality of evidence)*

1.9.4. 75 g of OGTT should be done with or without HbA1c. *(Moderate quality of evidence)*

1.9.5. If the OGTT cannot be performed, fasting plasma glucose and/or glycated hemoglobin (HbA1c) could be considered, though it has a significantly reduced accuracy. *(Moderate quality of evidence)*

1.9.6. Insulin levels should not be done to assay variability (depending on age, gender, and feeding status) and inaccuracy (absence of validated assay). *(Moderate quality of evidence)*

Summary of evidence: The evidence consistently shows an increased risk of hyperglycemia across all age groups which is independent of BMI with moderate quality of evidence. This warrants screening in both adolescents and adults with PCOS. For screening glucose intolerance either the WHO or ADA criteria is used.[15]

1. WHO criteria 2 hours 75 g OGTT
   - IGT 140–199 mg/dL
   - DM ≥200 mg/dL
2. ADA criteria fasting glucose level
   - IFG 100–125 mg/dL
   - DM ≥126 mg/dL

Usually done at diagnosis and repeated when the women are planning for a pregnancy or seeking fertility treatment.

Research gap: Given the practical and logistical considerations (time, inconvenience, cost, and accessibility) involved in performing OGTT for impaired glucose tolerance, T2D diagnosis, there is a clear need for further research to compare alternative diagnostic strategies against the OGTT, which may need to incorporate a combination of parameters, such as fasting glucose and HbA1c, to simplify glycemic evaluation in settings where regular OGTT may not be practical. There is an urgent need for a validated, easy-to-detect marker for assessing IR in PCOS.[15]

1.10. What is the risk in relatives?

Draft recommendations:

1.10.1. Healthcare professionals could consider that fathers and brothers of women with PCOS may have an increased prevalence of metabolic syndrome, type 2 diabetes mellitus, and hypertension. *(Moderate quality of evidence)*

1.10.2. Healthcare professionals, adults, and adolescents with PCOS, and their first-degree relatives should be aware of the increased risk of diabetes and the need for regular glycemic assessment. *(Moderate quality of evidence)*

1.10.3. The cardiometabolic risk in female first-degree relatives of women with PCOS remains inconclusive. *(Clinical practice point)*

Summary of evidence: Studies on PCOS have shown multiple relatives and siblings in families exhibiting autosomal dominant inheritance. When compared to first-degree relatives of controls, first-degree relatives of those with PCOS were more likely to suffer from metabolic syndrome, hypertension, diabetes, and PCOS though the quality of evidence is low. Subgroup analysis of these studies showed that the fathers and brothers of women with PCOS were more likely to suffer from metabolic syndrome, hypertension, and diabetes.[8] Some studies have shown that mothers and daughters of PCOS women are more likely to have PCOS, diabetes, hypertension, and metabolic syndrome, while others have negated this. Some studies have also looked into the siblings which showed a higher incidence of PCOS both in male and the females. The first-degree female relatives exhibited an increased prevalence of hyperandrogenism, menstrual irregularities, and ovarian morphological changes. Fathers of patients with PCOS had an increased risk of premature male pattern baldness (PMPB), and the DHEAS level was elevated in male first-degree relatives (FDRs).[16]

Research gaps: It becomes responsibility of clinicians to educate about the metabolic risk in relatives. Patient education booklets should be designed to create awareness. Recent studies looking specifically at sisters of women with PCOS did not find any significantly increased metabolic risks. More longitudinal studies with follow-up from infancy to adulthood are required to thoroughly capture the cardiometabolic risk for first-degree relatives of women with PCOS. Based on emerging evidence only, no routine recommendations are made for screening relatives in clinical practice.

CONCLUSION

Polycystic ovarian disease is a lifelong, enduring disease, and a common complex reproductive endocrinopathy with reproductive, metabolic, and mental health consequences. With a global prevalence of 9.2%, there is a difference in prevalence and clinical presentation among different ethnicities. All women with irregular menstruation should be further worked up for PCOS diagnosis. Rotterdam's criteria are the most recommended diagnostic method. According to the international guidelines if hyperandrogenism and irregular menstrual cycles are present an ultrasound polycystic morphology is not necessary for diagnosis. One should test all women with PCOS for metabolic abnormalities—OGTT and lipid profile, hypertension.

REFERENCES

1. The Rotterdam ESHRE/ASRM-sponsored PCOS consensus workshop group. Revised 2003 consensus on diagnostic criteria and long-term health risks related to polycystic ovary syndrome (PCOS). Hum Reprod. 2004;19(1):41-7.
2. Bharali M, Rajendran R, Goswami J, et al. Prevalence of polycystic ovarian syndrome in India: a systematic review and meta-analysis. Cureus. 2022;14(12):e32351.
3. Salari N, Nankali A, Ghanbari A, et al. Global prevalence of polycystic ovary syndrome in women worldwide: a comprehensive systematic review and meta-analysis. Arch Gynecol Obstet. 2024;310(3):1303-14.
4. Sharma M, Khapre M, Saxena V, et al. Polycystic ovary syndrome among Indian adolescent girls: a systematic review and metanalysis. Nepal J Epidemiol. 2021;11(3):1063-75.
5. Teede HJ, Misso ML, Costello MF, et al. Recommendations from the international evidence-based guideline for the assessment and management of polycystic ovary syndrome. Human reproduction. 2018;33(9):1602-18.
6. Yasmin A, Roychoudhury S, Paul Choudhury A, et al. Polycystic ovary syndrome: an updated overview foregrounding impacts of ethnicities and geographic variations. Life. 2022;12:1974.
7. Joham AE, Piltonen T, Lujan ME, et al. Challenges in diagnosis and understanding of natural history of polycystic ovary syndrome. Clin Endocrinol (Oxf). 2022;97:165-73.
8. Malik S, Jain K, Talwar P, et al. Management of Polycystic Ovary Syndrome in India. Fertil Sci Res. 2014;1:23-43.
9. Teede HJ, Tay CT, Laven JJ, et al. Recommendations from the 2023 international evidence-based guideline for the assessment and management of polycystic ovary syndrome. Eur J Endocrinol. 2023;189(2):G43-64.
10. Wang K, Li Y, Chen Y. Androgen excess: a hallmark of polycystic ovary syndrome. Front Endocrinol (Lausanne). 2023;14:1273542.

11. Christ JP, Cedars MI. Current Guidelines for Diagnosing PCOS. Diagnostics. 2023;13:1113.
12. Capuzzo M, La Marca A. Use of AMH in the Differential Diagnosis of Anovulatory Disorders Including PCOS. Front Endocrinol. 2021;11:616766.
13. Dewailly D, Gronier H, Poncelet E, et al. Diagnosis of polycystic ovary syndrome (PCOS): revisiting the threshold values of follicle count on ultrasound and of the serum AMH level for the definition of polycystic ovaries. Hum Reprod. 2011;26(11):3123-9.
14. Wild RA, Carmina E, Diamanti-Kandarakis E, et al. Assessment of cardiovascular risk and prevention of cardiovascular disease in women with the polycystic ovary syndrome: a consensus statement by the androgen excess and polycystic ovary syndrome (AE-PCOS) society. J Clin Endocrinol Metabol. 2010;95(5):2038-49.
15. Amisi CA. Markers of insulin resistance in polycystic ovary syndrome women: an update. World J Diabetes. 2022;13(3):129-49.
16. Shan D, Han J, Cai Y, et al. Reproductive health in first-degree relatives of patients with polycystic ovary syndrome: a review and meta-analysis. J Clin Endocrinol Metab. 2022;107(1):273-95.

2

CHAPTER

Lean versus Obese Polycystic Ovarian Syndrome

Vageesh Ayyar S, Madhuri Patil

BACKGROUND

Polycystic ovarian syndrome (PCOS) is a common metabolic and endocrine disorder seen in women during their reproductive age group. It is prevalent in about 10–15% of women worldwide during their fertile years. This syndrome is characterized by variety of symptoms and signs and the diagnostic criteria have evolved over the past three decades. About 70% of the PCOS women are obese and 30% are lean. There are ethnic differences in the prevalence of obese and lean PCOS which needs further elucidation. It usually presents with androgenic features and ovulatory dysfunction, which are more pronounced in the obese.[1] The prevalence of obesity is maximum in phenotype B. Women with PCOS have visceral adiposity when compared to age and BMI-matched controls and is a good measure of obesity even in lean PCOS. Testosterone promotes visceral fat accumulation and insulin resistance which in turn is a risk factor for metabolic and cardiovascular complications of PCOS. Insulin resistance reduces levels of SHBG and increases bioavailable androgens.

Subcutaneous and omental fat gene expression studies have shown an altered expression of genes related to obesity, insulin resistance, inflammation, and steroidogenesis. It is the epigenetic modification, which is linked to metabolic disease. Genetic and environmental factors have shown to affect human muscle and adipose tissue epigenetics.

2.1. What are nutritional and environmental influences throughout the life course and the perpetuation of the transgenerational inheritance of PCOS?

Draft recommendations:

2.1.1. Nutritional and environmental influences throughout the life course and the perpetuation of the transgenerational inheritance is seen in PCOS. *(Low quality of evidence)*

2.1.2. Poor quality diet, overnutrition, sedentary behavior, obesity, emotional stress, circadian rhythm disruption, poor gut health, or environmental chemical exposure (both intrauterine and after birth results in altered fetal programming with high risk of PCOS. *(Low quality of evidence)*

2.1.3 Genetic and epigenetic intrauterine growth programming results in a developmentally programmed thrifty genotype (obesity, premature adrenarche, and pubarche and metabolic syndrome) with activation of thrifty phenotype during childhood and adolescence that results in the development of PCOS in adulthood with increased risk of obesity, type II diabetes, metabolic syndrome, and fatty liver. *(Low quality of evidence)*

2.1.4. Obesity, IR, compensatory hyperinsulinemia along with chronic low-grade inflammatory state influence the clinical and metabolic parameters of PCOS. *(Clinical consensus statement)*

Summary of evidence: Children and adolescents born with intrauterine growth restriction (IUGR) should be followed closely for the development of adverse consequences, including pubertal problems and reproductive function abnormalities. Rapid weight gain in early life needs special attention in these children. Metabolic disorders, obesity, and cardiovascular risk factors which may start in childhood need close follow-up. Good nutrition and healthy lifestyle should be encouraged.[2]

Research gaps: Further studies on the genetic, epigenetic, metabolic, and environmental and endocrine aspects of IUGR are necessary. Unraveling the mechanism from fetal growth restriction to clinical and metabolic disturbances in women with PCOS will help in preventing the severity of PCOS.

2.2. Why are women with PCOS at increased risk of weight gain and Central Obesity?

Draft recommendations:

2.2.1. Visceral adiposity in PCOS is associated with increased IR, leading to exacerbation of reproductive and metabolic abnormalities. *(Low quality of evidence)*

2.2.2. Overeating, decreased physical activity, stress, developmental priming and epigenetics, and deficiency in magnesium, chromium, potassium, and vitamins E and C are responsible for visceral obesity. *(Clinical practice point)*

Summary of evidence: Obesity seen in more than two-thirds of women with PCOS. The highest incidence is seen in phenotype B followed by A and D. Women with phenotype C are least affected by obesity. The clinical heterogeneity and complex pathophysiology of PCOS has made understanding of relationship between excess fat, fat distribution and PCOS unclear. Central obesity increases insulin resistance and hyperandrogenism, which may exacerbate the clinical picture of PCOS.[3]

Research gaps: Rate of weight gain and excess weight/obesity causes considerable concern for PCOS women. Given the burden of obesity which exacerbates the clinical features of PCOS, prevention of weight gain through healthy lifestyle is vital.

2.3. How important is visceral obesity in pathogenesis and clinical manifestation of PCOS?

Draft recommendations:

2.3.1. Androgens influence visceral adiposity, which decreases adiponectin, induces leptin resistance and lipogenesis with high number of cortisol receptor in visceral adipose tissue that can result in increased cortisol response with increased activity of 5-α-reductase. *(Moderate quality of evidence)*

2.3.2. Visceral obesity results in metabolic and reproductive disturbances thus increases the manifestations of PCOS (insulin resistance, decreased insulin sensitivity, and increased dyslipidemia, ↑menstrual/ovulatory disturbances, ↑hyperandrogenism, ↓SHBG, ↓fertility and ↑pregnancy complications. *(High-quality of evidence)*

2.3.3. Visceral obesity results in neurohormonal activation and chronic inflammation which in turn increases the risk of metabolic syndrome. *(Moderate quality of evidence)*

2.3.4. It is recommended that screening women with PCOS for obesity by BMI and for visceral obesity by measuring waist circumference as it can influence the phenotype. *(Low quality of evidence)*

Summary of evidence: 60% PCOS women were overweight. A longitudinal study has shown that there is an 9% increased risk of PCOS for every 1 unit increase in BMI.[4] Hyperandrogenemia results in visceral obesity which in turn increases the hyperandrogenemia, due to reduced levels of SHBG and increased bioavailable androgens. Abdominal obesity is also associated with an increased testosterone production rate and a non-SHBG-bound androgen production. Obesity induced inflammation results in cascade of events leading to insulin resistance, dyslipidemia, increased ovarian androgen production, reproductive, and metabolic dysfunction.[6,7] There is also an important links between total and visceral body fat with insulin resistance, low-grade chronic inflammation, and circulating sex hormones.[8] Visceral obesity also reduces ART success, worsened psychological function, and increases risk of cardiovascular disease and DM2.

Research gaps: Visceral obesity may have an important impact on the early development of PCOS and obesity may change in degree and possibly in distribution from adolescence to postmenopausal age and these changes should be monitored.

2.4. Is lean PCOS also obese and why?

Draft recommendations:

2.4.1. Lean PCOS also has visceral adiposity with less muscle mass (Sarcopenic). *(Moderate quality of evidence)*

2.4.2. Sarcopenia adds to altered insulin function and manifestations of hyperandrogenism and metabolic disturbances in women with PCOS. *(Low-quality of evidence)*

2.4.3. Lean PCOS should be counseled regarding vigilance for progression to metabolic syndrome. *(Clinical practice point)*

2.4.4. Moderate physical activity and strength training exercise are recommended in women with lean PCOS to counter the metabolic issues associated with sarcopenia and PCOS. *(Moderate quality evidence)*

Summary of evidence: It has been well understood that PCOS is not exclusively seen in overweight or obese women. BMI is a poor measure of an individual's adipose-related disease burden. It is the fat quantity, quality, and location that matter. All women with PCOS have visceral adiposity as compared to age and BMI-matched controls thus present both in lean and obese PCOS. Therefore, it is not unusual to find a significant proportion of patients with normal BMI but having increased visceral fat. Visceral adipose tissue is important in providing information beyond other measures for obesity and for risk for the metabolic and cardiovascular complications of PCOS.[7] Many studies have shown that lean women with PCOS have more visceral obesity than control women with similar BMI and their metabolic risk is similar to obese women with PCOS.[9] Women with PCOS exhibit early signs of sarcopenia when compared to controls and probably this adds to altered insulin function and manifestations of hyperandrogenism and metabolic disturbances in PCOS.[8]

Research gaps: The long-term implications for metabolic syndrome in women with lean PCOS are still to be extensively studied. Why their metabolic and hormonal profiles are worse than women with similar BMI needs further understanding.

Data on sarcopenia in PCOS are sparse and conflicting. Evidence on sarcopenia in PCOS remains mixed and further research is warranted to clarify the influence of PCOS on sarcopenia.

2.5. Why are South Asians more prone to insulin resistance?

Draft recommendations:

2.5.1. South Asian Phenotype carries more fat with same BMI and have a higher risk of developing insulin resistance than other ethnic populations owing to evolution and genetic predisposition. *(Moderate quality of evidence)*

2.5.2. South Asians have more total and visceral fat with less lean mass, skeletal muscle, bone mineral density, and lower β-cell population compared to ethnic groups, which increase insulin resistance and further risk of metabolic syndrome. *(Moderate quality of evidence)*

Summary of evidence: Data suggest that South Asians are at high risk of developing insulin resistance (IR), even at low BMI. These data also suggest that South Asians have a higher risk of IR than other ethnic populations and normal-weight South Asians have higher risk than normal-weight people of other ethnic groups, including white and blacks which is related to abdominal/visceral obesity.[10] Probably evolutionary history of the South Asians has resulted in reduced β-cell mass and/or function coupled with low lean muscle mass, which may be responsible for IR. This is further complicated by ectopic fat stores in the liver and muscle, which results in IR.[11] Therefore, one must not waste muscles but activate them with exercise.

Research gaps: There is an urgent need to unravel the basic biological reasons and role of South Asian diets in development of poor insulin secretion, insulin resistance, and ectopic fat deposits that puts them at high risk of manifestations of insulin resistance.

2.6. What are the similarities and differences between lean and obese PCOS?

Draft recommendations:

2.6.1. Similar prevalence of acanthosis nigricans, menstrual dysfunction, hirsutism, and endometrial hyperplasia in both lean and overweight. *(Moderate quality of evidence)*

2.6.2. Hormonal profiles were also similar with respect to LH:FSH ratio, serum LH, progesterone and testosterone levels. *(Moderate quality of evidence)*

2.6.3. Both have insulin resistance and hyperinsulinemia with a prevalence of 83.3% and 93.1% in lean and overweight respectively. *(High quality of evidence)*

2.6.4. No difference between lean and obese on pelvic ultrasound features, viz., volume, AFC, and stroma. *(Moderate quality of evidence)*

2.6.5. Hormonal and metabolic imbalances are more frequently encountered in obese PCOS women. *(High quality of evidence)*

2.6.6. Android obesity, high triglyceride, and cholesterol levels are the only parameters that vary between obese and lean, being higher in obese PCOS. *(High quality of evidence)*

Summary of evidence: In each phenotype, it is important to distinguish an obese subphenotype which is associated with more severe metabolic issues and a mild subphenotype with normal bodyweight. Lean phenotype A PCOS patients tend to have more metabolic issues than other lean phenotypes but still have less metabolic issues than obese PCOS patients of phenotype B or C. Normoandrogenic phenotype D (OA + PCOM) has less severe endocrine and metabolic abnormalities.[5]

Table 1 gives salient differences between obese and lean PCOS.[12]

TABLE 1: Salient differences between obese and lean PCOS.

Lean PCOS	***Obese PCOS***
LH, GH↑	IGF↑ IGFBP-1↓
> Ovulatory	> Anovulatory
Ovarian vol↑	Peak E2 concentrations↓
Metabolic syndrome↓	Metabolic syndrome↑
Insulin R↓	Insulin, androgens↑, SHBG↓ insulin R↑
DM and HT	IGT and DM↑
GDM	Leptin↑
	Dyslipidemias↑

Research gaps: Identifying the pathogenetic mechanisms which make lean PCOS women more prone to certain manifestations is essential. The contribution of visceral fat to the phenotypical presentations also needs to be studied.

2.7. Is obesity associated with greater reproductive dysfunction?

Draft recommendations:

2.7.1. Obesity is associated with menstrual dysfunction and can lead to precocious menarche (<9 years), irregular cycles, and oligo-/amenorrhea. *(High quality of evidence)*

2.7.2. Obesity is also associated with sexual dysfunction—difficulty of performance and impairment of desire, arousal, and orgasm. *(Low quality of evidence)*

2.7.3. Incidence of infertility is three times higher in obese PCOS. *(High quality of evidence)*

2.7.4. Obesity influences treatment of infertility with poor response to fertility drugs, requirement for higher dose of gonadotropins, altered endometrial function, lower success rates with ART due to altered ovarian responsiveness and oocyte quality and decreased oocytes retrieved and a higher incidence of cancellation of cycle. *(High quality of evidence)*

2.7.5. Implantation, clinical pregnancy rate (CPR), and live birthrate (LBR) progressively worsen with increasing BMI with a higher incidence of miscarriage rate. *(High quality of evidence)*

2.7.6. BMI >29 kg/m^2 is associated with reduced success of ongoing pregnancy and a 4% lower pregnancy rate per kg/m^2 BMI increase. *(Moderate quality of evidence)*

2.7.7. Obesity in PCOS results in increased time to conception. *(Low quality of evidencc)*

Summary of evidence: Obesity disrupts the hypothalamic-pituitary-gonadal axis, resulting in either anovulation or luteal phase defect, consequently reducing amounts of progesterone. The mechanisms resulting in chronic anovulation in PCOS may not be linked exclusively to metabolic alterations like insulin resistance.[5]

Obesity is also linked to alterations in the granulosa cells of the ovary and its secretions around the oocyte. There are variations in follicular fluid contents such as insulin, triglycerides, free fatty acids, proinflammatory cytokines, oxidized low-density lipoprotein, and fatty acid composition. Obesity is usually associated with hyperinsulinemia and insulin resistance with increased ovarian androgen production. Obesity promotes insulin resistance and complicates PCOS symptoms.[5]

Obesity has been linked to anovulation, decreased ovarian response to ovulatory prescription medications, changed oocyte and endometrial activity, an elevated risk of fertility problems, and reduced rates of live birth following IVF.[13] The risk of miscarriage, gestational diabetes mellitus, gestational hypertension, preeclampsia, cesarean section, preterm birth, fetal growth restriction, and low birthweight are higher in women with PCOS and are probably independent of BMI.[14]

Research gaps: Our understanding about metabolically healthy obesity is as yet incomplete. The contribution of visceral obesity to reproductive function is still being understood.

2.8. What is the treatment for lean and obese PCOS?

Draft recommendations:

2.8.1. Assessment with an interdisciplinary team taking into consideration BMI and other chronic conditions is essential. *(Moderate quality of evidence)*

2.8.2. Lifestyle changes are beneficial for weight loss, maintaining weight and building muscle mass in both obese and lean PCOS. *(High quality of evidence)*

2.8.3. Therapeutic interventions such as combined oral contraceptives, antiandrogens, and insulin sensitizers are helpful in treating symptoms related to anovulation, hyperandrogenemia, and insulin resistance. *(High quality of evidence)*

2.8.4. Metformin, an insulin sensitizer, was more successful in restoring menstruation (55%) and ovulation (45%) in lean women with PCOS compared with their obese counterparts. *(Moderate quality of evidence)*

2.8.5. 3 g/day of myoinositol appeared to have a positive effect on lean women with PCOS, which led to reductions in luteinizing hormone, androgen levels, "high-sensitivity C-reactive protein" and facilitated insulin tolerance. *(Very Low quality of evidence)*

2.8.6. Suppression of ovarian androgen production using oral contraceptive preparations, Androgen receptor blockers [cyproterone acetate, flutamide, spironolactone, and 5-α-reductase inhibitors (finasteride)] and cosmetic treatment (hair removal by electrolysis or laser therapy is useful to reduce hair growth. *(High quality of evidence)*

2.8.7. Mild and moderate cases of acne may respond to topical preparations such as benzylperoxide and/or clindamycin or retinoid creams, whereas severe cases may need additional oral treatment with a tetracycline group of antibiotics and in some cases oral isotretinoin. *(Low quality of evidence)*

2.8.8. Progesterone therapy protects the endometrium in both lean and obese PCOS. *(Moderate quality of evidence)*

2.8.9. There is no evidence of a beneficial impact of short-term weight loss on LBR after IVF treatment or pregnancy outcome. *(Low quality of evidence)*

2.8.10. Surgical techniques such as unilateral or bilateral laparoscopic ovarian drilling was found to be associated with comparable rates of successful pregnancies between lean and obese PCOS. *(Moderate quality of evidence)*.

2.8.11. Bariatric surgery may be an option in women with a BMI of >35 kg/m^2 and the presence of comorbidities. Bariatric surgery does not improve the clinical live birthrate in women with PCOS and high BMI. *(Moderate quality of evidence)*

2.8.12. In obese women, lifestyle modification previous to IVF does not enhance embryo utilization or cumulative live birth rate. The duration it takes to lose weight may not be beneficial in combating the problems of declining ovarian reserve. *(Moderate quality of evidence)*

2.8.13. Lean women with PCOS exhibited a significantly higher rate of fertilization compared with their overweight counterparts (BMI ≥25 kg/m^2). *(Low quality of evidence)*

Summary of evidence: Metabolic, hormonal, and hematological derangements exist in both lean and obese although these are equal or less obvious in thin PCOS as compared to obese PCOS. Insulin resistance is inherent in PCOS regardless of BMI and should be managed early on. Results are promising in terms of managing the lean phenotype more than obese PCOS. Lifestyle modifications, restoration of ovulation with the use of pharmacological interventions, and even IVF in refractory cases can provide symptomatic relief and increase the chances of successful pregnancy both in Lean and Obese PCOS Women.[15] Obesity has been linked to anovulation, decreased ovarian response to ovulatory prescription medications, modified oocyte and endometrial activity, and an elevated risk of infertility with reduced birth rates following IVF. Lean women with PCOS have exhibited a significantly greater rate of fertilization compared with their overweight counterparts.[16] One cannot refuse infertility treatment to obese patients, especially in the presence of medical comorbidities and shared decision-making procedures should be initiated, trying to balance the patient's autonomy with normal efficiency.

Various management options are available for lean PCOS. Even though weight loss is not considered important in lean PCOS women, it may help to improve the metabolic parameters and reproductive function. Lean PCOS women should aim to maintain their weight and increase muscle mass. Lifestyle modification by diet and exercise has shown improved insulin resistance and hyperandrogenism. Metformin therapy is more useful in restoring ovulatory cycles in lean PCOS when compared to obese women.

Research gaps: Results from recent literature should be interpreted with caution as various limitations were apparent with regard to the study designs. The sample size was often too small and Rotterdam criteria were not uniformly used for the diagnosis of PCOS.

CONCLUSION

It is apparent that metabolic and hormonal derangements do exist in lean PCOS. However, these are either equal or less compared to obese PCOS. Insulin resistance is inherent in PCOS regardless of bodyweight. Certain manifestations like hyperandrogenism are more prevalent in lean PCOS. When it comes to management, results are promising in terms of managing the lean PCOS but well-designed RCTs are lacking in lean PCOS.

The challenge of the overweight patient:

- Risk of inappropriate treatment:
  - Weight loss effective in many patients
  - Problems in pregnancy
- Risks of IVF and stimulation:
  - Under-response to FSH
  - Difficulty in imaging ovaries
  - Difficulty in anesthesia
  - Difficulty in embryo transfer
- Risk of pregnancy:
  - Congenital abnormality
  - Gestational diabetes and hypertension
  - Delivery either vaginal or abdominal
  - Risks to immediate and future health of the child

The challenge of the thin patient is as follows:

- Risk of inappropriate treatment:
  - Weight gain before pregnancy and correction of nutrition
  - Ovulation induction before IVF

- Risk of IVF and stimulation:
  - Over-response to FSH
  - May need additional LH or hCG in follicular phase
  - Lack of response to GnRH agonist trigger
  - Risk of OHSS
- Risk of pregnancy:
  - Poor fetal growth
  - Higher perinatal mortality

Therefore, one must assess individuals and couples systematically for lifestyle, weight, smoking, stress, medical issues and drug intake and genetic factors as well as environmental risks factors. One needs to provide advice and opportunity to correct these by offering programs to reduce risks to offspring.

REFERENCES

1. Escobar-Morreale HF. Polycystic ovary syndrome: definition, aetiology, diagnosis and treatment. Nat Rev Endocrinol. 2018;14(5):270-84.
2. Darendeliler F. IUGR: Genetic influences, metabolic problems, environmental associations/triggers, current and future management. Best Pract Res Clin Endocrinol Metabol. 2019;33:101260.
3. Satyaraddi A, Cherian KE, Kapoor N, et al. Body composition, metabolic characteristics, and insulin resistance in obese and nonobese women with polycystic ovary syndrome. J Hum Reprod Sci. 2019;12:78-84.
4. Teede HJ, Joham AE, Paul E, et al. Longitudinal weight gain in women identified with polycystic ovary syndrome: results of an observational study in young women. Obesity. 2013;21(8):1526-32.
5. Carmina E, Lobo RA. Comparing lean and obese PCOS in different PCOS phenotypes: evidence that the body weight is more important than the rotterdam phenotype in influencing the metabolic status. Diagnostics. 2022;12:2313.
6. Glueck C, Goldenberg N. Characteristics of obesity in polycystic ovary syndrome: etiology, treatment, and genetics. Metabolism. 2019;92:108-20.
7. Lear SA, Humphries KH, Kohli S, et al. Visceral adipose tissue accumulation differs according to ethnic background: results of the Multicultural Community Health Assessment Trial (M-CHAT). Am J Clin Nutr. 2007;86(2):353-9.
8. Dadachanji R, Patil A, Joshi B, et al. Elucidating the impact of obesity on hormonal and metabolic perturbations in polycystic ovary syndrome phenotypes in Indian women. PLoS One. 2021;16(2):e0246862.
9. Elnashar A. Lean polycystic ovary syndrome: a narrative review. Clin Exp Obstet Gynecol. 2024;51(6):142.
10. Deepa R, Sandeep S, Mohan V. Abdominal obesity, visceral fat and type 2 diabetes. Asian Indian Phenotype. 2007:138-52.
11. Vitek W, Hoeger K, Legro RS. Treatment strategies for infertile women with polycystic ovary syndrome. Minerva Ginecologica. 2016;68:450-7.
12. Silfen ME, Denburg MR, Manibo AM, et al. Early endocrine, metabolic, and sonographic characteristics of polycystic ovary syndrome (PCOS): comparison

between nonobese and obese adolescents. J Clin Endocrinol Metabol. 2003;88(10):4682-8.

13. Elnashar AM. Update on obesity and assisted reproductive technology. Middle East Fertil Soc J. 2023;28(1).
14. Bahri Khomami M, Shorakae S, Hashemi S, et al. Systematic review and meta-analysis of pregnancy outcomes in women with polycystic ovary syndrome. Nature communications. 2024;15(1):5591.
15. Toosy S, Sodi R, Pappachan JM. Lean polycystic ovary syndrome (PCOS): an evidence-based practical approach. J Diab Metabol Disord. 2018;17:277-85.
16. Misra A, Khurana L, Isharwal S, et al. South Asian diets and insulin resistance. Br J Nutr. 2009;101:465-73.

CHAPTER 3

Screening and Management of Mental Health in Polycystic Ovary Syndrome

Uday Thanawala, Madhuri Patil

INTRODUCTION

Polycystic ovary syndrome (PCOS) is a common and distressing endocrine disorder associated with lower quality of life (QoL), subfertility, diabetes, cardiovascular disease, depression, anxiety, eating disorders, and can potentially influence sexual function. The etiology of PCOS involves a complex mixture of genetic, hormonal, and lifestyle factors that contribute to its pathophysiology and the associated mental health challenges. Stress, in various forms, including metabolic, inflammatory, oxidative, and emotional, is identified as a significant contributor to the pathogenesis of PCOS.

Many physicians are aware of the symptoms such as menstrual disturbance, infertility, and aspects of metabolic syndrome, but the mental disarray which this disorder, can potentially cause, is often overlooked.

3.1. What is the prevalence and severity of reduced quality of life?

Draft recommendations:

3.1.1. PCOS has adverse impact on quality of life in adults. *(Moderate quality of evidence)*

3.1.2. All PCOS women should be asked about their perception of PCOS symptoms, in particular, impact on quality of life, and what are the key concerns and priorities for the management of their symptoms. *(Clinical practice point)*

Summary of evidence: The prevalence of reduced quality of life is very variable in the populations studied in different parts of the world. Though the clinical features of PCOS are reported, much is not reported on the emotional well-being.[1] In several studies, lower psychological health scores have been reported. There is an increasing incidence of anxiety and depression. One must adapt a PCOS questionnaire to score for emotional well-being. The polycystic ovary syndrome questionnaire (PCOSQ) has 26 items and includes emotions, body hair, weight, infertility and menstrual abnormalities and the modified polycystic ovary syndrome questionnaire (MPCOSQ) adds acne.[1,2] In adolescents, the Pediatric Quality of Life Inventory (PedsQL) questionnaires have been applied in PCOS.[3] The study had high degree of heterogeneity and did not show much difference in the psychological well-being of adolescents with PCOS and controls of the same age.

Research Gaps: Quality of life is reduced in women with PCOS but most publications have a high degree of heterogeneity, challenges, and differences with appropriate tools used and the populations studied were diverse. Moreover, the QoL is also influenced by sociocultural factors.

Despite this it is important to formally measure QoL in women with PCOS. There were large gaps in adequate data being published in the adolescent group. Moreover, the role of MPCOSQ in clinical settings is unclear as the key factors in QoL are controversial.

3.2. What is the prevalence and severity of anxiety and depression?

Draft recommendations:

3.2.1. The clinician should be aware of the high prevalence of anxiety symptoms and disorders and moderate to severe depressive symptoms and depression in adults and adolescents with PCOS. *(Strong quality of evidence)*

3.2.2. All clinicians should screen both adolescents and adult women for depression using regionally validated screening tools. *(Strong quality of evidence)*

3.2.3. If moderate or severe depressive or anxiety symptoms are detected, the patient should be further assessed, counseled and, if necessary, referred to a psychologist or psychiatrist for appropriate treatment. *(Strong quality of evidence)*

3.2.4. The screening for anxiety and depression should ideally be done at the time of diagnosis of PCOS with repeat screening if necessary. No fixed interval is recommended and reassessment should be based on clinical judgment, risk factors, comorbidities and life events. *(Clinical practice point)*

3.2.5. Screening for mental health disorders comprises assessment of risk factors, symptoms, and risk of deliberate self-harm and suicidal intent. *(Clinical practice point)*

Summary of evidence: Polycystic ovary syndrome is a chronic disorder causing problems such as infertility, cosmetic issues, and obesity. Obesity, in turn, leads to bodyimage issues and sleep apnea. The constant pressure of compliance with treatment and frustrating results raises the anxiety and depression, impacting the QoL;[1] which in turn can then influence compliance with lifestyle and medical management.

Anxiety and depression are both common among PCOS. The prevalence of depression in women with PCOS is high and ranges from 16 to 55%. The most frequently observed signs and symptoms of depression in women with PCOS are fatigue, sleep disorders, and low mood. Suicidal thoughts and attempts are less frequently observed, although their probability was sevenfold higher than in the control group.[4]

According to a study done in Kashmir in 2015—among women with PCOS—About 23% of cases had major depressive disorder as compared to 7.5% of controls, 1.8% had dysthymia, 15.45% had panic disorder compared to 5% of controls, 6.36% had obsessive compulsive disorder compared to 2.5% of controls, 8% cases had suicidality, 2.72% of cases were bipolar affective disorder, and 15.45% had generalized anxiety disorder (GAD).[5]

It is also a known fact that hormonal treatment in PCOS women can influence the mood of the women.

Screening: Guidelines from different countries vary on recommending routine screening for common mental health disorders for all adults and adolescents, particularly with chronic physical health problems and in the perinatal period. Moreover, mental health guidelines in most countries generally do not recognize PCOS as a condition with a high risk of depression and anxiety.[6] This is especially true in a country like India where awareness of patients and physicians is low and psychological illness is considered taboo.

Research gaps: Routine screening for depressive and anxiety symptoms though recommended is not done in all patients. The absence of screening can influence the treatment as well as to provide opportunities to improve well-being and QoL. Routine screening can be influenced by time, resources available and access to screening tools. The international screening tools may not be appropriate for our population and we need to create one for our country looking at the different socio-cultural backgrounds. One should also remember that overdiagnosis can increase distress in these women as it adds to another potentially stigmatizing diagnosis.

3.3. What is the prevalence and severity of body image distress?

Draft recommendation:

3.3.1. Clinicians should be aware that features of PCOS can have a negative impact on body image. *(Strong quality of evidence)*

Summary of evidence: Body image is defined as the mental picture of one's body, an attitude about the physical self, appearance, and state of health, wholeness, normal functioning, and sexuality. Body image is a component of a larger concept of self that for women includes feeling feminine and attractive, enjoying one's body as a symbol of social expression, and as a way of being in the world.

Polycystic ovary syndrome has a higher prevalence of negative body image than the controls. This negative body image can subsequently impact the thoughts and feelings about health, appearance, QoL, mood, and physical fitness.[1] It is the excess weight, hirsutism and acne, and anxiety and depression along with sociocultural factors that influence body image.[1,7] When we assess body image, consider body dissatisfaction, signs, and symptoms of excess androgens (hirsutism and acne), disordered eating, waist hip ratio, and weight. The assessment of body image disorders can be done by different methods of psychometric analyses. There are limited meta-analyses on this subject.

Age is an important factor affecting perception of one's body. Women below the age of 25 years have a higher difficulty with accepting their appearance. The widespread idolization of thinness leads to negative body image among women with normal bodyweight.[8]

Research gaps: Assessment of body image disorders should be a part of comprehensive screening in PCOS women. Negative body image in PCOS appears to be increased and may result in increased depression and poorer QoL. We still do not have screening and assessment tools that are easy to use and widely applicable and are therefore needed. Keeping in mind several symptoms of PCOS, women may require extensive screening tools that may then become burdensome both for the patient and doctor and may not be performed. Therefore, it is important to individualize the screening in those who need it, as screening in all may have resource implications and increase time of consultation.

3.4. What is the prevalence and severity of psychosexual dysfunction?

Draft recommendations:

3.4.1. Though exact prevalence not known, PCOS women present with variable psychosexual dysfunction that influence fertility, mood disorders, and require medications. *(Low quality of evidence)*

3.4.2. Clinicians should discuss psychosexual function with couples which may be related to their psychological condition. *(Low quality of evidence)*

Summary of evidence: Psychosexual dysfunction refers to sexual problems or difficulties that have a psychological origin, based on cognitions and/or emotions such as depression, low self-esteem, and negative body image.[1,9] As the prevalence of psychosexual dysfunction is increased in PCOS women, it may impact QoL and relationships with the spouse. Moreover, the use of oral contraceptives, anti-androgens and fertility drugs can also affect psychosexual function in PCOS women as well as the general population.[1] Most studies that looked at psychosexual function had a low to moderate risk of bias. Most studies did not show much difference between PCOS women and the general population, but the PCOS women did have a lower total sexual function, lubrication, orgasm, and satisfaction after the sexual act.[1] Lower sexual function may be related to negative body image due to excessive weight, hirsutism, and greater difficulties in engaging in social contact due to appearance.

Research gaps: Women with PCOS score lower on psychosexual function questionnaires than those who do not have PCOS. As most studies did not explore related distress with psychosexual disorders, there is limited evidence on the interpretation of a connection between the two and, therefore, the clinical relevance is unclear. No evidence points out the relationship between psychosexual dysfunction and the presence of infertility, higher weight, and other factors. Screening and assessment may be considered in sexually active women to offer appropriate intervention to optimize sexual function and improve quality of life. Future studies assessing psychosexual distress scores are needed for stronger evidence.

3.5. What is the prevalence and severity of eating disorders?

Draft recommendations:

3.5.1 Eating disorders including anorexia nervosa; bulimia nervosa and binge-eating disorder should be enquired in all PCOS patients irrespective of the weight as these are common and may influence management. *(Low quality of evidence)*

3.5.2. If eating disorders are suspected, further assessment with appropriate management should be offered. *(Clinical practice point)*

Summary of evidence: Eating disorders are clinically significant and may be related to behavioral (e.g., binging, and excessive restriction), cognitive (e.g., excessive dietary restraint and negative body image) and emotional features.[1,2] Eating disorders have a higher prevalence in PCOS and can affect health, QoL, and social interaction.[2] This warrants an increased awareness to diagnose the condition in PCOS women which could then result in effective assessment and management of the condition. Several studies have reported the risk of at least one eating disorder including bulimia nervosa, binge eating disorder, anorexia nervosa, or night eating syndrome in adults with PCOS compared to controls.[1] These studies reported a higher incidence of eating disorders in PCOS compared to non-PCOS adults. Most studies included adults and not adolescents so the incidence in adolescents is unknown or not reported.

Research gaps: Women with PCOS have a higher prevalence of eating disorders and face negative biopsychosocial consequences experiencing many of the identified risk factors for eating disorders. Many adult women and most adolescents with eating disorders are undiagnosed and unaware of the disorder. Therefore, increased awareness and consideration of assessment and diagnosis are important. Due to the complexity of the disorder, screening and treating is a major challenge. Routine screening is not recommended as the current tools available are not satisfactory and the assessment may be influenced by resources available and there also could be constraints of time. When suspected, there should be heightened awareness for screening and managing.

3.6. What are the different psychological and therapeutic options that can be offered for the management and support of depression and/or anxiety or disordered eating?

Draft recommendations:

3.6.1. Clinicians should provide tailored information, education and information resources that is high-quality, culturally appropriate and inclusive to all with PCOS in a timely, respectful and empathic manner. *(Moderate quality of evidence)*

3.6.2. A multidisciplinary approach for counseling and screening is necessary involving trained clinicians who could apply evidence-based knowledge for counseling. *(Low quality of evidence)*

3.6.3. Appropriate time should be given during the consultation, which helps shared decision-making for further management options. *(Low quality of evidence)*

3.6.4. Women with disordered eating, body image distress, low self-esteem, or psychosexual dysfunction should be offered Psychological therapy *(cognitive behavioral therapy)* as first-line management besides additional antianxiolytics and antidepressant medications if deemed necessary in adults where anxiety and depression are clearly documented and those with suicidal tendency. *(Low quality of evidence)*

3.6.5. Overlooking management of anxiety and depression may impact adherence to PCOS treatment to improve overall QoL. *(Clinical practice point)*

Summary of evidence: Psychosocial function as measured by PedsQL in two studies showed that the total quality of life was lower in women with PCOS as compared to women without PCOS though it did not reach statistical significance.[1] Cultural issues, including those issues related to fertility and stigma of having PCOS, have a great sociocultural impact, but have not looked at the role of families especially in adolescence in improving interpersonal relationships. Lack of patient-healthcare provider interactions, support, empathy, and shared decision-making make PCOS care deficient.[10] Supportive therapies like cognitive behavioral therapy, behavioral therapy, and interpersonal therapy are available for the treatment of psychological conditions associated with PCOS which result in clinically significant improvements in mental health with improvement in quality of life and psychosocial well-being.[11] A psychotherapist can deliver better care to PCOS women depending on age, diagnosis, severity of symptoms, and available resources.

The supportive therapies have been shown to improve the condition and associated distress and impairment with consequent improvement in self-esteem and body image.

A study by Jiskoot G, et al. found a large effect of cognitive behavioral therapy on psychological symptoms.[12] Major depressive disorder anxiety disorder, panic disorder, and phobias which occur in a small percentage of PCOS women can be treated by antidepressants and anxiolytics respectively, though their role and efficacy is unclear. There was a single small study that showed the efficacy of antidepressants. Thus, the evidence for the use of antidepressants and anxiolytics is of low quality.[13]

Research gaps: Inconsistent care of PCOS women was seen due to a lack of priority, limited education, and awareness of the clinician. There were clear gaps seen in evidence-based information provision at the time of diagnosis and ongoing treatment. There is hardly any data from developing countries on information resources, models of care, available models, and cultural and linguistic considerations. Most data are from developed countries, which may not apply to India. Even studies from developed countries had low to moderate risk of bias. In developed countries we do have some form of structural lifestyle management, cardiometabolic risk assessment or management of reproductive health, but management of emotional well-being screening and management is lacking.

Psychological treatment is usually guided by the results of systematic reviews and meta-analyses where available, or where they are not available high-quality RCTs and evidence-based guidelines for the treatment of body image distress, self-esteem, or feminine identity as there are no accepted guidelines present. Lifestyle and other therapies that target PCOS features have also shown improvement in psychological symptoms in PCOS. Limited available research suggests that cognitive behavioral therapy is effective in the treatment of body image distress, self-esteem, feminine identity, or psychosexual dysfunction. Thus, there is need for further research in this area. The recommendation for the use of antidepressants and anxiolytics is basically based on general population guidelines for the treatment of anxiety and depression.

CONCLUSION

Thus, it is not only the presenting symptom of the patient which needs to be tackled, but today the physician must asertain the mental well being of a PCOS woman and address it appropriately.

We need to deal with two aspects when it comes to mental health:

1. Physicians being aware of the various disorders that can be present—body image, depression, anxiety, psychosexual disorders, eating disorders, and difficulty in losing weight, sleep apnea leading to fatigue.
2. Disorders like anxiety and depression should be routinely screened in all PCOS women—with appropriate screening tools.

Many such tools are available—WHO-5 wellbeing index being the simplest and others more detailed ones like, PHQ9 or PCOSQ which consists of 26 items measuring five aspects of Health-Related Quality of Life: Emotions, body hair, weight, infertility problems, and menstrual problems. Choose any screening tool—which you feel your patients will comply and fill. Evaluate the score and if you find the score is in the danger zone of moderate to severe depression/anxiety—do not hesitate to refer for evaluation with a mental health expert.

In the clinic—listening to the patient, kind words, and encouragement (TLC—tender loving care) will go a long way in improving the mental status of these patients and managing this complex condition effectively.

REFERENCES

1. Teede HJ, Tay CT, Laven JJ, et al. Recommendations from the 2023 international evidence-based guideline for the assessment and management of polycystic ovary syndrome. Eur J Endocrinol. 2023;189(2):G43-64.
2. Dokras A, Stener-Victorin E, Yildiz BO, et al. Androgen Excess-Polycystic Ovary Syndrome Society: position statement on depression, anxiety, quality of life, and eating disorders in polycystic ovary syndrome. Fertil Steril. 2018;109(5):888-99.
3. Çoban ÖG, Tulacı ÖD, Adanır AS, et al. Psychiatric disorders, self-esteem, and quality of life in adolescents with polycystic ovary syndrome. J Pediatr Adolesc Gynecol. 2019;32:600-4.
4. Dybciak P, Raczkiewicz D, Humeniuk E, et al. Depression in polycystic ovary syndrome: a systematic review and meta-analysis. J Clin Med. 2023;12(20):6446.
5. Hussain A, Chandel RK, Ganie MA, et al. Prevalence of psychiatric disorders in patients with a diagnosis of polycystic ovary syndrome in Kashmir. Indian J Psychol Med. 2015;37(1):66-70.
6. Malhi GS, Bassett D, Boyce P, et al. Royal Australian and New Zealand College of Psychiatrists clinical practice guidelines for mood disorders. Aust N Z J Psychiatry. 2021;55(1):7-117.
7. Alur-Gupta S, Chemerinski A, Liu C, et al. Body-image distress is increased in women with polycystic ovary syndrome and mediates depression and anxiety. Fertil Steril. 2019;112:930-8.e1.
8. Sioma-Markowska U, Milena O. Polycystic ovary syndrome and the perception of body image by women. Gin Pol Med Project. 2021;59(1):028-034.
9. Clayton AH, Goldstein I, Kim NN, et al. The International Society for the Study of Women's Sexual Health Process of Care for Management of Hypoactive Sexual Desire Disorder in Women. Mayo Clin Proc. 2018;93(4):467-87.
10. Dokras A, Saini S, Gibson-Helm M, et al. Gaps in knowledge among physicians regarding diagnostic criteria and management of polycystic ovary syndrome. Fertil Steril. 2017;107:1380 6.e1.
11. Brutocao C, Zaiem F, Alsawas M, et al. Psychiatric disorders in women with polycystic ovary syndrome: a systematic review and meta-analysis. Endocrine. 2018;62:318-25.
12. Jiskoot G, van der Kooi AL, Busschbach J, et al. Cognitive behavioural therapy for depression in women with PCOS: systematic review and meta-analysis. Reprod Biomed Online. 2022;45:599-607.
13. Masoudi M, Ansari S, Kashani L, et al. Effect of sertraline on depression severity and prolactin levelsin women with polycystic ovary syndrome: a placebo-controlled randomized trial. Int Clin Psychopharmacol. 2021;36:238-43.

CHAPTER 4

Lifestyle Management

4.1 DIET AND NUTRITION

Shilpa Joshi, Shefali Bhardwaj

INTRODUCTION

Polycystic ovary syndrome (PCOS) is a multidimensional endocrine disorder affecting a substantial proportion of women world over. PCOS management requires a multidisciplinary approach addressing the symptoms and signs along with the lifestyle aspects that contribute to this condition. Latest research findings have highlighted the critical role of lifestyle interventions including diet, exercise, and psychological care that play an important role in improvement of several health outcomes. However, the efficacy of these interventions varies based on cultural, social, and individual factors. This document delivers evidence-based recommendations for lifestyle and dietary interventions personalized to the unique needs of Indian women with PCOS, emphasizing the importance of a personalized and patient-centric approach.

4.1.1. Are lifestyle interventions effective for improving anthropometric, metabolic, reproductive, fertility, quality of life, and emotional well-being outcomes?

Draft recommendations:

4.1.1.1. Lifestyle intervention (exercise alone or multicomponent diet combined with exercise and behavioral strategies) should be recommended for all women with PCOS, to improve anthropometric, metabolic, reproductive, fertility, quality of life, and emotional well-being outcomes. *(Strong quality of evidence)*

4.1.1.2. Every individual with PCOS should undergo a thorough assessment of their lifestyle, including diet, exercise, sleep patterns, emotional well-being, stress levels (both work-related and personal), and current quality of life. *(Clinical Consensus)*

4.1.1.3. To facilitate this, a standardized and user-friendly questionnaire should be developed, enabling patients to provide information to healthcare professionals for effective interpretation. *(Clinical practice point)*

4.1.1.4. Interventions should be delivered by a multidisciplinary team that includes a dietitian, physiotherapist, psychologist, besides clinicians ensuring a holistic approach to care. *(Clinical practice point)*

4.1.1.5. Healthcare providers should create a personalized lifestyle prescription tailored to the specific needs and circumstances of individuals. *(Clinical practice point)*

Summary of evidence: Polycystic ovary syndrome has a high prevalence and adverse impact of excess weight on the symptoms of PCOS, and efficacy of lifestyle interventions in PCOS was an important component in the management of PCOS. Recent studies suggest the positive impact of lifestyle interventions on improving anthropometric, metabolic, quality of life, and emotional well-being outcomes.[1,2] The impact of these interventions on reproductive and fertility outcomes is limited and inconclusive.[3]

Research gaps:

1. There is a lack of high-quality, large-scale RCTs specifically focusing on Indian women with PCOS.
2. Research is needed to explore how cultural and social factors influence the effectiveness of lifestyle interventions in this population.
3. Also, longitudinal studies will be beneficial to see long-term effects of the same.

4.1.2. What are the dietary interventions that are effective for improving anthropometric, metabolic, reproductive, fertility, quality of life, and emotional well-being outcomes?

Draft recommendations:

4.1.2.1. A personalized energy deficit should be prescribed for women requiring weight loss, depending on individual energy requirements, bodyweight, and physical activity levels. *(Clinical practice point)*

4.1.2.2. Women with PCOS should be advised to follow a hypocaloric diet rich in whole grains, lean proteins, healthy fats, and low glycemic index foods. Reducing the intake of refined carbohydrates and sugars is crucial. *(Clinical practice point)*

4.1.2.3. Including anti-inflammatory foods and traditional Indian spices like turmeric and fenugreek may offer additional benefits. *(Clinical practice point)*

4.1.2.4. Including nuts and oil seeds as sources of good quality fats and protein will compensate for the reduction in carbohydrates. *(Clinical practice point)*

Summary of evidence: Recent studies highlight the effectiveness of low glycemic index diets, Mediterranean diets, and anti-inflammatory foods in improving metabolic and reproductive outcomes. These dietary patterns have been associated with significant improvements in insulin sensitivity, lipid profiles, and menstrual regularity.[4-6] The use of traditional Indian spices with anti-inflammatory properties has also been shown to be beneficial.[7]

Research gaps:

1. More studies are required to explore the effectiveness of culturally tailored dietary interventions for Indian women with PCOS, including the role of traditional Indian dietary practices.
2. From the research, the guidelines that can be followed across the HCPs are needed. Some evolving research on the effectiveness of seed cycling in the management of PCOS is being established. However, large RCT data is lacking, and more research is needed. Seed cycling is a new holistic healthcare practice for PCOS in which the person, during their follicular phase (day 1–15), consumes 1–2 teaspoons of raw, freshly ground flax seed and pumpkin seeds. Later in the luteal phase (days 15–28) 1–2 teaspoons of raw, freshly ground sunflower and sesame seeds are recommended.[8]
3. The effectiveness of an Indianized "Mediterranean like" diet for the Indian population is needed to increase diet compliance due to familiarity, taste, and cost constraints.

4.1.3. How would you counsel the women with PCOS regarding diet for maintaining the weight?

Draft recommendations:

4.1.3.1. The concept of "diet" needs to be changed to a "healthy eating pattern" as the word "diet" is perceived to be something very restrictive and generates a sense of deprivation among people and a perception that they cannot follow it for long. *(Clinical practice point)*

4.1.3.2. Dietary counseling for women with PCOS should emphasize the importance of a balanced diet, portion control for creating negative calorie balance, and regular meal timings. Counseling should focus on the benefits of low glycemic index foods, high fiber intake, and regular physical activity. Behavioral strategies like mindful eating and keeping a food diary should also be encouraged. *(Clinical practice point)*

4.1.3.3. Counseling should emphasize on making "healthy eating" as a pattern for the entire family as these dietary changes are good for the entire family's metabolic health. *(Clinical practice point)*

4.1.3.4. Dietitians with optimal knowledge of eating habits should be involved in counseling. *(Clinical practice point)*

4.1.3.5. Women with PCOS should be counseled for a lifelong focus on diet for weight loss and prevention of further weight gain. *(Clinical practice point)*

4.1.3.6. For those who are not overweight, they should be counseled to focus on a healthy lifestyle which includes diet and exercise to prevent excess weight gain. *(Clinical practice point)*

Summary of evidence: Studies highlight the positive impact of hypocaloric, low carbohydrate, high glycemic index, and anti-inflammatory diet.[4-6] The need for adequate training of healthcare professionals who manage adolescents and women with PCOS is necessary. They should have an empathetic approach to develop realistic lifestyle management goals and have a broader focus beyond weight.

Research gaps:
1. Limited data exist on the effectiveness of culturally specific counseling strategies for Indian women.
2. Future research should focus on how traditional dietary patterns can be modified and optimized for weight management in this population.
3. Also, it is imperative to notice that compliance with diet is affected by behavioral therapy tools and the identification of emotional eating practices. Research in this area is also important.

4.1.4. Barriers to weight loss?

Draft recommendations:

4.1.4.1. Weight loss for women with PCOS should be approached as a collaborative effort between the patient and a multidisciplinary team of healthcare professionals (HCPs), including clinicians, dietitians, exercise physiologists, and mental health specialists. *(Clinical practice point)*

4.1.4.2. A coordinated and one-stop solution that integrates medical, nutritional, psychological, and exercise support is crucial for effective management. *(Clinical practice point)*

4.1.4.3. Patient-centric approach, tailored to the individual's unique needs, is more effective than generalized guidelines. *(Clinical practice point)*

4.1.4.4. Delivering scientific facts and knowledge in an empathetic manner to improve motivation. *(Clinical practice point)*

4.1.4.5. Support groups help to create awareness among patients and family members alike. *(Clinical practice point)*

Summary of evidence: The challenges of PCOS management fall into four categories: (1) The weakness of clinical evidence, (2) low compliance to the management of PCOS, (3) hurdles faced by healthcare professionals, and (4) the influence of culture and social environment.[9] Cognitive behavior therapy (CBT) has shown a positive impact in women with PCOS toward decreasing anxiety, improving quality of life in women with hirsutism, and increasing compliance and rate of pregnancy. Cognitive behavioral therapy (CBT) is a form of psychotherapy that alters cognitive patterns for behavioral rearrangement to modify psychological indications and behaviors.[10]

Research gaps:

1. More research is needed to explore the most effective strategies for overcoming barriers to weight loss in women with PCOS.
2. Research focusing on the unique barriers faced by Indian women with PCOS is limited.
3. Studies should investigate how cultural, social, and economic factors influence weight loss efforts and how to effectively address these barriers within the Indian context and Indian sensibility/sensitivities.

CONCLUSION

Effective management of PCOS needs to be comprehensive and personalized. By focusing on personalized lifestyle interventions, including culturally appropriate dietary modifications, regular physical activity, and psychological support, the health outcomes and quality of life for women with PCOS can significantly be improved. It is crucial to identify the unique barriers faced by Indian women in PCOS management and develop approaches that address these challenges within the cultural and social framework of the population. Further research is required to support these recommendations and ensure that they are effective for and manageable by the women with PCOS in India as well as the healthcare providers.

REFERENCES

1. Abdolahian S, Tehrani FR, Amiri M, et al. Effect of lifestyle modifications on anthropometric, clinical, and biochemical parameters in adolescent girls with polycystic ovary syndrome: a systematic review and meta-analysis. BMC Endocrine Disorders. 2020;20:1-7.
2. Zhao K, Nie L, Ye X, et al. Effects of mind-body interventions on polycystic ovary syndrome: a comprehensive meta-analysis. J Ovarian Res. 2024;17(1):154.
3. Espinós JJ, Solà I, Valli C, et al. The effect of lifestyle intervention on pregnancy and birth outcomes on obese infertile women: a systematic review and meta-analysis. Int J Fertil Steril. 2020;14(1):1.
4. Le ST, Haubrick K. The comparison of the DASH, Hypocaloric, Mediterranean/Low Glycemic Diet/Low Carbohydrate, as a nutritional intervention in polycystic ovary syndrome in overweight women: a systematic review. J Food Studies. 2021;10(1):37.
5. Porchia LM, Hernandez-Garcia SC, Gonzalez-Mejia ME, et al. Diets with lower carbohydrate concentrations improve insulin sensitivity in women with polycystic ovary syndrome: a meta-analysis. Eur J Obstet Gynecol Reprod Biol. 2020;248:110-7.
6 Shang Y, Zhou H, He R, et al. Dietary modification for reproductive health in women with polycystic ovary syndrome: a systematic review and meta-analysis. Front Endocrinol. 2021;12:735954.

7. Sharma N, Kumar V, Langeh U, et al. A review on the pharmacological potential of Indian spices in polycystic ovarian syndrome. J Reprod Health Med. 2023;4:1-5.
8. Zafar M, Rabail R, Bibi S, et al. Seed cycling: approach for polycystic ovarian syndrome. Food Human. 2024:100274.
9. Guan M, Li R, Wang B, et al. Healthcare professionals' perspectives on the challenges with managing polycystic ovary syndrome: a systematic review and meta-synthesis. Patient Educ Counsel. 2024;123:108197.
10. Tang R, Yang J, Yu Y, et al. The effects of cognitive behavioral therapy in women with polycystic ovary syndrome: a meta-analysis. Front Psychol. 2022;13:796594.

4.2 EXERCISE AND YOGA

Ulka A Natu, Vibhuti Rao, Smitha Moorthy

INTRODUCTION

Insulin resistance is one of the main features of PCOS and exercise is known to reduce insulin resistance. The first step in the management of PCOS is weight reduction with changes focused on lifestyle management, diet, and exercise.[1] Physical activity is defined as any bodily movement generated by the skeletal muscles which results in energy expenditure. Exercise is a physical activity that is planned, structured and repetitive, which is often undertaken to improve or maintain health, well-being, and/or performance. Yoga is not just a routine exercise; it is rather a form of mind-body intervention. Cultivation of correct psychological attitudes is of high significance when we think of incorporating yoga as a therapy. Yoga has a bifold technique, physical as well as psychological. No physical exercise alone would contribute to harmony when carried out in state of physical agitation. Influence of mind over body is more than that of body over mind. Therefore, yoga practice with respect to its physical and psychophysiological viewpoint is important to correct the pathogenesis of PCOS.

4.2.1. What are the components one needs to look at when recommending exercise and yoga to women with PCOS?

Draft recommendations:

4.2.1.1. An initial assessment for comorbidities, current physical activity, eating habits and disorders, and quality of life is necessary. Subsequently, anthropometric and cardiovascular risk assessment (waist circumference, BMI, and blood pressure) and exercise tolerance (cardiorespiratory fitness, muscle strength, exercise capacity, and physical limitations) need to be evaluated using validated self-administration questionnaires. *(Clinical practice point)*

4.2.1.2. Assessment and reassessment of cardiorespiratory fitness and muscular strength, power, and endurance, may be effective strategies to increase exercise self-efficacy given their responsiveness to exercise interventions, particularly among those who are physically inactive or exercise-naïve. *(Clinical practice point)*

4.2.1.3. Yoga therapy can be a preferred choice to incorporate into a patient's daily routine to optimize other lifestyle interventions and treatments. *(Clinical practice point)*

4.2.1.4. There is a lack of evidence supporting any one type and intensity of exercise to improve anthropometric, metabolic, hormonal, and reproductive or psychological outcomes. *(Moderate quality of evidence)*

Summary of evidence: The exercise professional should prioritize assessments that are available to them while being considerate of their resources and expertise.[1] In those with higher weight, weight management can be associated with significant clinical improvements and the following key points need to be considered: A lifelong focus on the prevention of further weight gain if the goal is to achieve weight loss, a tailored energy deficit could be prescribed for women, considering individual energy requirements. The body weight and physical activity levels have a value in improvement of central adiposity (e.g., waist circumference and waist-hip ratio) or metabolic health the need for ongoing assessment and support. Published studies did not show much difference in the outcome between high-intensity interval training versus moderate-intensity continuous training.[1]

No ideal drug or method has been discovered so far in science which would destroy or neutralize the offending factors alone, but would not harm other normal tissues. Efficiency of organs/cooperation between different systems cannot be brought by mere ingestion of medicines. The training of organs and systems is done directly or indirectly by yoga, incorporating yogic practices as yoga therapy.[2] Mind plays an important role even in the genesis of PCOS. Psychophysiological disturbances, every emotion, especially negative disturbances interfere with the tonic rhythm of muscles and vessels and can also result in disturbance in breathing.

Research gap: These recommendations are based on international evidence-based guidelines and need to be explored in the Indian population. Due to the social, cultural, and genetic factors, the Indian population require a more comprehensive assessment before suggesting high-intense exercises. Moreover, published studies did have low risk of bias.

4.2.2. Are exercise interventions effective for improving anthropometric, metabolic, reproductive, fertility, quality of life, and emotional well-being outcomes?

Draft recommendations:

4.2.2.1. The available evidence, including mechanistic studies, shows that exercise interventions can improve a variety of cardiometabolic health outcomes in PCOS, including insulin sensitivity, central obesity, and cardiorespiratory fitness. *(Low quality of evidence)*

4.2.2.2. Exercise intervention can improve quality of life and emotional well-being. *(Low quality of evidence)*

4.2.2.3. Exercise has been shown to improve central adiposity and reduce cardiovascular disease risk. *(Clinical practice point)*

4.2.2.4. Yoga therapy may significantly decrease menstrual irregularity, clinical hyperandrogenism, fasting blood glucose, fasting insulin, and homeostatic model assessment-insulin resistance value. *(Low quality of evidence)*

Summary of evidence: Exercise has been widely studied for its effects on cardiometabolic health in women with PCOS.[3] Evidence consistently shows that exercise modestly improves waist circumference, a marker for visceral fat. While fasting insulin levels generally improve, changes in lipid profiles, body weight, and fasting blood glucose are inconsistent. Exercise, especially when combined with diet, is more effective than minimal intervention in improving insulin sensitivity. Meta-analyses indicate that aerobic exercise, whether moderate-intensity continuous training (MICT) or high-intensity interval training (HIIT), can improve cardiorespiratory fitness by about one metabolic equivalent (~3.5 mL/kg/min).[4] Patten et al. in their study found that HIIT leads to better improvement in cardio-metabolic and reproductive outcomes than moderate-intensity training in women with PCOS.[5] In women with PCOS, exercise reduces free androgen levels by increasing SHBG, which binds to testosterone, and lowers hyperinsulinemia, positively affecting ovarian function. Exercise also benefits mental health, reducing symptoms of stress, depression and anxiety and improving quality of life.[6,7] For women with PCOS and mental health concerns, combining exercise with psychological treatment may offer greater benefits. A systematic review and meta-analyses by Verma et al.[8] found that yoga therapy may significantly decrease menstrual irregularity, clinical hyperandrogenism, fasting blood glucose, fasting insulin, and homeostatic model assessment-insulin resistance value. Additionally, a scoping review of meditation and mindfulness supports the potential role of yoga beyond an exercise routine. Patil et al.[9] in their pilot study found that a 12-week yoga intervention helps in an overall improvement in anthropometric, hormonal, biochemical, ovarian morphology, and infertility-related QoL parameters compared to the control group.

Research gap: Exercise is a first-line treatment for women with PCOS, but research is limited by heterogeneity in study designs, including differences in intervention length, modality, intensity, and participant diversity. While some studies align with physical activity guidelines, few meet recommendations for significant health benefits or meaningful weight loss (5–10% of body weight).

Additionally, the impact of exercise on mental health and quality of life in PCOS is under-researched. The low strength of evidence suggests the need to conduct well-designed RCTs to assess the efficacy of yoga therapy for PCOS.

4.2.3. Is exercise also important in Lean PCOS?

Draft recommendations:

4.2.3.1. Physical activity is important for lean PCOS women with a focus on a healthy lifestyle and prevent weight gain. *(Clinical practice point)*

4.2.3.2. Lean PCOS have low muscle mass thus, strength training exercises and low-impact yoga practice would be beneficial. *(Clinical practice point)*

4.2.3.3. Yoga and meditation have an effective role in managing day-to-day stress levels and psychological health. *(Clinical practice point)*

Summary of evidence: Even though women with lean PCOS may not struggle with weight issues, they can still experience other symptoms like insulin resistance, hormonal imbalances, and menstrual irregularities, all of which can be improved with regular physical activity. Early mechanistic studies support the role of exercise in improving insulin sensitivity and restoring mitochondrial physiology.[3] Additionally, exercise can support mental well-being and improve quality of life by reducing symptoms of anxiety and depression, which are often associated with PCOS.

Yoga, pilates, and tai chi are examples of mind-body workouts that can not only burn calories but also lower stress levels, which can increase PCOS symptoms. For strength training to increase muscular mass, one can use resistance bands, weights, or your body weight.

Research gap: We found no RCT investigating the role of exercise in lean PCOS. Many questions are still unanswered. More studies that consider weight training, diet, and specific macronutrient to improve are necessary PCOS symptoms. Moreover, most studies look at the effect of exercise and diet in obese PCOS than lean PCOS women. Thus, further studies are warranted to investigate the benefits of exercise interventions in lean women with PCOS.

4.2.4. What exercise would you advise for obese and lean PCOS?

Draft recommendations:

4.2.4.1. For both obese and lean PCOS, a balanced exercise regimen is beneficial, although the regimen may need individualization. *(Clinical practice point)*

4.2.4.2. Any physical activity consistent with population guidelines will have health benefits and within this, healthcare professionals should advise sustainable physical activity based on individual preferences and goals. *(Low quality of evidence)*

4.2.4.3. All adults should undertake physical activity as doing some physical activity is better than none. Adults should limit the amount of time spent being sedentary (e.g., sitting and screen time) as replacing sedentary time with physical activity of any intensity (including light intensity) provides health benefits. *(Clinical practice point)*

4.2.4.4. For the prevention of weight gain and maintenance of health, adults (18–64 years) should aim for a minimum of 150–300 minutes of moderate-intensity or 75–150 minutes of vigorous intensity aerobic activity per week or an equivalent combination of both spread throughout the week, plus muscle-strengthening activities (e.g., resistance/flexibility) on two nonconsecutive days per week. *(Low quality of evidence)*

4.2.4.5. For the promotion of greater health benefits, including modest weight loss and prevention of weight regain, adults (18–64 years) should aim for a minimum of 250 minutes of moderate-intensity or 150 minutes of vigorous-intensity aerobic activity per week or an equivalent combination of both spread throughout the week, plus muscle-strengthening activities (e.g., resistance/flexibility) on two nonconsecutive days per week. *(Low quality of evidence)*

4.2.4.6. Adolescents should aim for at least 60 minutes of moderate-to-vigorous—intensity physical activity per day, including activities that strengthen muscle and bone, at least three times per week. *(Low quality of evidence)*

4.2.4.7. For patient who prefers yoga therapy can practice 10 minutes of meditation and 20 minutes of dynamic asana postures under a trained yoga therapist five times a week. *(Low quality of evidence)*

Summary of evidence: There is limited evidence to support one type or intensity of exercise over another for improving anthropometric, metabolic, hormonal, reproductive, or psychological outcomes in women with PCOS. A systematic review and meta-analyses by Colombo et al.[10] found no significant differences between high-intensity interval training (HIIT) and moderate-intensity continuous training (MICT) in these outcomes, with low or very low certainty of evidence. However, one study indicated HIIT may be more effective than MICT for improving menstrual regularity. Comparisons between HIIT and resistance training, as well as diet + MICT versus diet + MICT + resistance training, also showed no significant differences.

Research gap: There are currently insufficient RCTs comparing different exercise modalities in individuals with PCOS to determine whether one form of exercise is superior to another for managing the condition.

4.2.5. How would you counsel women with PCOS regarding Exercise and Yoga for maintaining weight?

Draft recommendations:

4.2.5.1. Counseling should involve motivational interviewing, questions directed at barriers in weight loss, and identifying which barriers are crossed with ease which are moderate and which are extremely difficult. *(Clinical practice point)*

4.2.5.2. Patients have to come out with a commitment to start with minor changes, to begin with, and a time-bound plan to attempt to cross major barriers. *(Clinical practice point)*

4.2.5.3. Identify support systems at home/work/social media. *(Clinical practice point)*

4.2.5.4. Referral to trained allied healthcare professionals may help in optimizing physical activity. *(Clinical practice point)*

4.2.5.5. Journaling changes *(Clinical practice point)*

4.2.5.6. Reporting to mentor *(Clinical practice point)*

Summary of evidence: When promoting physical activity, exercise professionals should consider an individual's cultural and socioeconomic circumstances, personal preferences, comorbidities, physical capacity, and overall management goals. Effective counseling involves positive psychology, motivational interviewing, active listening, and open-ended questions, empowering individuals to take responsibility for self-care and behavior change. Health practitioners have to provide a nonjudgmental, shame-free environment, avoiding weight-stigmatizing beliefs and attitudes that may unconsciously influence lifestyle recommendations.[11] Respecting personal preferences, including a desire not to discuss weight, is crucial. Weight-neutral approaches, such as mindful eating, body image work, and building self-esteem, can achieve similar outcomes as traditional dietary therapies over 12 months while fostering sustainable healthy behaviors.

Research gap: Studies from India are needed to help to define components of counseling for women to promote exercise and yoga. Yoga is very popular among Indian women, hence, there are chances that women will accept yoga therapy as a potential mind-body intervention to manage PCOS.

4.2.6. What are the barriers to weight loss?

Draft recommendations:

4.2.6.1. Barriers to weight loss are similar to barriers to lifestyle changes in general. *(Clinical practice point)*

4.2.6.2. The difficulty in achieving and sustaining weight loss in PCOS can be attributed to a variety of physiological, psychological, and socioeconomic factors. *(Low quality of evidence)*

4.2.6.3. Key barriers to weight loss can be at individual-level (e.g., time and financial pressure, psychological comorbidities, and lack of motivation for maintaining a healthy lifestyle), treatment-related (e.g., high cost and long duration of treatment, and no relief of symptoms), system-level (e.g., lack of professional support and empathy, and unavailability of allied health professionals), and environmental barriers (e.g., lack of social support and exercise environment), insulin resistance, and hormonal imbalance can make weight loss difficult. *(Low quality of evidence)*

4.2.6.4. Regular follow-ups are necessary at weekly intervals, for 3 months. Then at monthly intervals for 6 months and then every 3 months thereafter. *(Clinical practice point)*

4.2.6.5. At 3 months intervals, it is important to evaluate them on patient-reported outcomes such as quality of life and levels of sleep quality and anxiety. *(Clinical practice point)*

Summary of evidence: Barriers and facilitators to optimize engagement and adherence to physical activity should be discussed, including psychological factors (e.g., body image concerns, fear of injury, fear of failure, and mental health), personal safety concerns, environmental factors, physical limitations, socioeconomic factors, sociocultural factors, and personal motivators for change. The value of broader family engagement should be considered. Referral to suitably trained allied healthcare professionals needs to be considered for optimizing physical activity in women with PCOS. Self-monitoring including fitness tracking devices and technologies for step count and exercise intensity could be considered as an adjunct to support and promote active lifestyles and minimize sedentary behaviors. Healthcare professionals should be aware of their weight biases and the impact this has on their professional practice and women with PCOS. Health policymakers, managers, and educators should promote awareness of weight stigma and invest in weight stigma education and minimization strategies.

The findings of Guan et al.[12] state that the barriers to weight loss from the perspective of health professionals can be categorized as the weakness of clinical evidence; women's low adherence to PCOS management; various obstacles that healthcare professionals face; and the influence of social environment and culture. Healthcare professionals should be aware of weight-inclusive practices that promote acceptance of and respect for body size diversity and focus on the improvement of health behaviors and health outcomes for people of all sizes. In PCOS this includes: acknowledging that while higher weight is a risk factor for PCOS and its complications, it is only one indicator of health and broader factors should be assessed asking permission to discuss and measure weight and using strategies to minimize discomfort (e.g., blind weighing) recognizing that the terms "overweight" and "obese/obesity" can be stigmatizing with suggested alternatives including "higher weight". It is important to explain how weight information will be used to inform risks prevention and treatment and how not knowing may impact on the recommendations. One must tailor lifestyle modification according to individual goals and preferences offering all women best practice assessment, treatment and support regardless of weight, acknowledging that weight may be a nonmodifiable risk factor when using lifestyle modification alone.

Research gap: Limited qualitative research has explored barriers to weight loss in women with PCOS. Weight management in Indian patients has social and cultural implications. Studies are needed to explore barriers to weight loss from an Indian perspective for sustainable and clinically meaningful weight loss.

CONCLUSION

To encourage every PCOS to exercise, it should be made cost-effective and easily accessible. One can reach out to many by making it available at community centers, sporting grounds/facilities, with ease of access in groups and with minimal equipment. One could further reduce the cost by making available electronic health apps that can be easily viewed on the mobile phone, which practically everyone possesses. In case the PCOS woman is unable to lose weight and has insulin resistance, one should consider the involvement of exercise specialists or physiotherapists for structured exercise regimens, which will help in reducing and maintaining weight. The involvement of a dietician to provide an appropriate diet helps further in weight loss programs. The benefit is maximum of exercise and nutrition when it is under close supervision of an expert.

REFERENCES

1. Teede HJ, Tay CT, Laven JJ, et al. Recommendations from the 2023 international evidence-based guideline for the assessment and management of polycystic ovary syndrome. Eur J Endocrinol. 2023;189(2):G43-64.
2. Rao VS, Armour M, Cheema BS, et al. Use of traditional and complementary medicine by ethnic Indian women living with polycystic ovary syndrome: a global survey. BMC Complementary Med Therap. 2023;23(1):392.
3. Sabag A, Patten RK, Moreno-Asso A, et al. Exercise in the management of polycystic ovary syndrome: a position statement from Exercise and Sports Science Australia. J Sci Med Sport. 2024.
4. Breyley-Smith A, Mousa A, Teede HJ, et al. The effect of exercise on cardiometabolic risk factors in women with polycystic ovary syndrome: a systematic review and meta-analysis. Int J Environment Res Pub Health. 2022;19(3):1386.

5. Patten RK, McIlvenna LC, Levinger I, et al. High-intensity training elicits greater improvements in cardio-metabolic and reproductive outcomes than moderate-intensity training in women with polycystic ovary syndrome: a randomized clinical trial. Hum Reprod. 2022;37(5):1018-29.
6. Singh B, Olds T, Curtis R, et al. Effectiveness of physical activity interventions for improving depression, anxiety and distress: an overview of systematic reviews. Br J Sports Med. 2023;57(18):1203-9.
7. Toval A, Bakker E, Granada-Maia J, et al. Effects of physical exercise on health-related quality of life in coronary heart disease patients: a systematic review and meta-analysis. Eur J Prevent Cardiol. 2023;30(Suppl 1):zwad125.239.
8. Verma A, Upadhyay V, Saxena V. Effect of yoga therapy on health outcomes in women with polycystic ovary syndrome: a systematic review and meta-analysis. Am J Lifestyle Med. 2023;17(1):73-92.
9. Patil AD, Pathak SD, Kokate P, et al. Yoga intervention improves the metabolic parameters and quality of life among infertile women with polycystic ovary syndrome in Indian population. Int J Yoga. 2023;16(2):98-105.
10. Colombo GE, Dafauce Bouzo X, Patten RK, et al. Comparison of selected exercise training modalities in the management of PCOS: a systematic review and meta-analysis to inform evidence-based guidelines. JSAMS Plus. 2023;2:100024.
11. Colombo GE, Pirotta S, Sabag A. Diet and exercise in the Management of Polycystic Ovary Syndrome: practical considerations for person-centered care. Semin Reprod Med. United States: Thieme Medical Publishers, Inc.; 2023.
12. Guan M, Li R, Wang B, et al. Healthcare professionals' perspectives on the challenges with managing polycystic ovary syndrome: a systematic review and meta-synthesis. Patient Educ Counsel. 2024;123:108197.

4.3 BEHAVIORAL STRATEGIES FOR POLYCYSTIC OVARY SYNDROME

Rutvi Manish Pandya, Nehal Manish Pandya, Manish R Pandya

INTRODUCTION

The polycystic ovarian syndrome (PCOS) is a common condition affecting women across their entire lifespan with significant physiological, metabolic, reproductive, and psychological sequelae. Numerous studies have found an increased prevalence of anxiety and depression among women with PCOS. The psychological sequelae can disrupt social, family, and interpersonal relationships in the social domain. The complete psychological impact and its management however has not yet been elucidated. The inclusion of behavioral and psychological strategies including goal setting, self-monitoring, and cognitive behavior therapy (CBT) can help to improve these symptoms. A positive effect has been seen on quality of life with social and family support as it reduces stress, increases confidence, provides a sense of security, and improves interpersonal relationship.

4.3.1. What is the effect of PCOS on the psychological well-being and personality of women?

Draft recommendations:

4.3.1.1. Psychological well-being is severely impacted in women with PCOS causing significant morbidity. *(Clinical practice point)*

4.3.1.2. All PCOS women should be questioned to assess traits such as impulsivity, reward-seeking behavior, self-control, and conscientiousness. *(Clinical practice point)*

4.3.1.3. Those women showing signs of anxiety or depression should be offered lifestyle interventions, psychotherapy, and if needed medical treatment. *(Strong recommendation but low quality of evidence)*

Summary of evidence: Polycystic ovarian syndrome results in psychological morbidity such as depression, poor body image and self-esteem, loss of feminine identity, poor psychosexual function, and reduced quality of life.[1]

A number of studies have shown higher rates of depression and anxiety in women with PCOS compared to the general population independent of body weight and a shared genetic component between depression and PCOS has been found. Personality traits are features that influence mood, thoughts, and behavior, and are stable over time. Personality traits such as impulsivity and sensitivity to reward have been identified as risk factors for weight gain, while self-control and conscientiousness are protective against it.[2] Evaluation of these traits can help to identify patients that might benefit from lifestyle intervention. These steps go a long way in planning a holistic and comprehensive approach for PCOS management.

Research gap: Whether these personality and behavioral traits are a cause or the sequelae of PCOS are uncertain. There is a paucity of studies on the effect on the psychological well-being of women with PCOS.

4.3.2. Can behavior modification interventions aid in the management of PCOS?

Draft recommendations:

4.3.2.1. The clinician should be aware of the various behavior modification interventions that can be offered to women with PCOS. *(Clinical Practice point)*

4.3.2.2. Behavior modification interventions help to optimize psychological and emotional well-being of women suffering from PCOS. *(Clinical Practice point)*

4.3.2.3. Behavioral strategies such as goal setting, self-monitoring, problem-solving assertiveness training, reinforcing changes, and relapse prevention to optimize weight management, healthy lifestyle, and emotional well-being in women with PCOS. *(Moderate quality of evidence)*

4.3.2.4. They must be counseled to improve adherence to and sustainability of other measures taken for the management of PCOS like diet, exercise, and pharmacotherapy. *(Clinical Practice point)*

Summary of evidence: Behavioral interventions (e.g., goal setting, peer-group support, self-monitoring, stimulus control, problem solving, assertiveness training, and slower eating) can help to reinforce lifestyle changes, reduce relapses, and optimize weight management, and emotional wellbeing of women with PCOS.[3] Behavioral and cognitive interventions are required to improve sustainability of lifestyle changes, through considering not only the specific behavior, but also their antecedents, consequences, and cognition.[4]

Psychosocial interventions such as cognitive behavioral therapy, acceptance and commitment therapy, mindfulness-based stress reduction combined with lifestyle modifications, or multicomponent behavioral modification program were found to improve depression, quality of life (QOL), fatigue or sleep issues, self-esteem, body image, perceived stress, mindfulness, and negative affect in women with PCOS.[5]

Research gap: Limited studies that are heterogenous and with moderate quality of bias have been published. There is paucity of evidence to definitively support implementation of behavioral therapy in addition to lifestyle management in PCOS women. Further randomized controlled trials are needed to evaluate the specific role of behavior modification interventions in the management of PCOS.

4.3.3. What is the utility of mindfulness programs in managing PCOS?

Draft recommendations:

4.3.3.1. Integration of meditation with conventional treatment modalities of management in PCOS women may improve QoL. *(Clinical practice point)*

4.3.3.2. Mindfulness interventions may improve psychosocial well-being and QoL in women with PCOS and therefore can be used as an adjunct to conventional treatment in women with PCOS. *(Clinical practice point)*

4.3.3.3. Meditation and mindfulness-based healthy lifestyle may improve psychological and metabolic parameters in PCOS women. *(Very low quality of evidence)*

4.3.3.4. Depression Anxiety Stress Scales (DASS-21) scale should be used to monitor the psychological distress in patients. *(Low quality of evidence)*

Summary of evidence: Meditation and mindfulness techniques are a clinical application of principles involving the key element of nonjudgmental acceptance of psychological distress thereby reducing the tendency to ruminate over these experiences. They promote stress alleviation due to an enhanced relaxation response, improve glycemic control, and decrease depression as well as anxiety. DASS-21 (Depression, Anxiety, and Stress scales) scores were found to be significantly lower in PCOS women after implementation of mindfulness stress management program.[6]

Practice of meditation and mindfulness on a regular basis have reported positive effects. It has helped in reducing stress, depression and anxiety, improved sleep and mood and also had a positive effect on metabolic symptoms like hypertension and abnormal sugar levels.

Research gap: Researchers are still exploring the impact of mindfulness on psychological and other symptoms in women with PCOS. Large sample size and long-term follow-up are needed to validate the impact of mindfulness techniques in PCOS.

4.3.4. What is the role of cognitive behavioral therapy in the management of PCOS?

Draft recommendations:

4.3.4.1. Cognitive behavioral therapy (CBT) has well-characterized benefits in, improving the patient's quality of life. *(Low quality of evidence)*

4.3.4.2. Cognitive behavioral therapy helps in alleviating diseases associated with depression, anxiety, and obesity that can help in improving quality of life in women with PCOS. *(Low quality of evidence)*

4.3.4.3. Clinicians should screen PCOS patients for psychological distress and refer those positive to a psychiatrist for cognitive behavioral therapy. *(Clinical practice points)*

Summary of evidence: Cognitive behavioral therapy (CBT) is the first-line psychological treatment that modifies cognitive patterns and provides behavioral restructuring to alter psychological symptoms and behaviors. CBT is effective in lowering depression scores and anxiety in women with PCOS thus improving QoL.

In CBT, one needs to assess negative automatic thoughts, cognitive distortions (jumping to conclusions, selective abstraction, and arbitrary inference), assumptions, feelings, and core beliefs. CBT involves techniques like thought record, Socratic questioning, examining evidence, thought replacement, and behavioral experiences. A multidisciplinary team which includes endocrinologists, psychologists, dieticians, gynecologists, endocrine-specialized nurses improve the outcome of CBT. It should include a minimum of 8-weekly sessions and three family-based sessions.

Use of CBT exhibited obvious advantages in the alleviation of anxiety and improvement of QoL in hirsutism. It also improves compliance and pregnancy rates in patients with PCOS.[7]

Research gap: There is insufficient evidence to demonstrate the effectiveness of CBT as published studies have methodological differences and bias. More *clinical trials* are needed to assess how many sessions of CBT are necessary to treat depression in women with PCOS. Higher-quality studies are needed to clarify the role of CBT in PCOS and to assess how many sessions of CBT are necessary to treat depression in women with PCOS.[7]

4.3.5. What is the consensus regarding use of traditional, complementary, and integrative medicine (TCIM) in PCOS?

Draft recommendations:

4.3.5.1. TCIM approaches may play an important role in the ongoing treatment regimen to help to provide culturally sensitive patient-centred care. *(Clinical practice point)*

4.3.5.2. Yoga helps to improve overall health of women with PCOS. *(Clinical practice point)*

4.3.5.3. One on one or group yoga sessions specifically tailored for PCOS should be encouraged and organized. *(Clinical practice point)*

4.3.5.4. TCIM can be used for symptoms that are not managed by current medical approaches *(Clinical practice point)*

Summary of evidence: Till date, there have been limited studies on the use of TCIM in women with PCOS. A global survey from 2023 found the prevalence of TCIM use among PCOS women to be 80%. Yoga and Ayurveda were the most frequently practiced TCIM modalities with a prevalence of 57% and 37%, respectively. Yoga was primarily used to improve overall health, manage weight, stress, hormonal imbalance, and emotional well-being.[8]

The use of TCIM is largest among Asians due to deeply rooted cultural values, a recommendation from family/friends, dissatisfaction with the current medical approach, perception of TCIM being natural and safe, and the quest for holistic health.

Research gap: Reasons for not using TCIM include inadequate information, uncertainty about effectiveness, and not being prescribed by their doctor. A lot more to be done to provide safe and evidence-based TCIM practices in terms of the exchange and transformation of knowledge between the health practitioners of different modalities, and the need for the right infrastructure and skills to deliver the best care to these women.

CONCLUSION

In our battle with PCOS, "the whole is greater than the sum of its parts". Adjunctive use of behavioral strategies in the armamentarium against PCOS is the need of the hour. The optimal complexity, intensity, and behavioral components of lifestyle interventions for women with PCOS need to be addressed to make management more comprehensive and successful. Strategies targeting improved motivation, social support, and psychological well-being should be focused upon. There is accumulating evidence that supports holistic approaches, such as meditation and mindfulness, in improving psychological well-being and QoL outcomes.

REFERENCES

1. Pitchai P, Sreeraj SR, Anil PR. Awareness of lifestyle modification in females diagnosed with polycystic ovarian syndrome in India: explorative study. Int J Reprod Contracept Obstet Gynecol. 2016;5(2):470-6.
2. Oberg E, Lundell C, Blomberg L, et al. Psychological well-being and personality in relation to weight loss following behavioral modification intervention in obese women with polycystic ovary syndrome: a randomized controlled trial. Eur J Endocrinol. 2020;183(1):1-11.
3. Al Wattar BH, Hussain NM, Khan KS. Lifestyle interventions in women with polycystic ovary syndrome: a scoping systematic review of randomised evidence. Medicina de Familia. SEMERGEN. 2022;48(3):186-94.
4. Cowan S, Lim S, Alycia C, et al. Lifestyle management in polycystic ovary syndrome–beyond diet and physical activity. BMC Endocr Disord. 2023;23(1):14.
5. Phimphasone-Brady P, Palmer B, Vela A, et al. Psychosocial interventions for women with polycystic ovary syndrome: a systematic review of randomized controlled trials. F&S Rev. 2022;3(1):42-56.
6. Stefanaki C, Bacopoulou F, Livadas S, et al. Impact of a mindfulness stress management program on stress, anxiety, depression and quality of life in women with polycystic ovary syndrome: a randomized controlled trial. Stress. 2015;18(1):57-66.
7. Tang R, Yang J, Yu Y, et al. The effects of cognitive behavioral therapy in women with polycystic ovary syndrome: a meta-analysis. Front Psychol. 2022;13:796594.
8. Rao VS, Armour M, Cheema BS, et al. Use of traditional and complementary medicine by ethnic Indian women living with polycystic ovary syndrome: a global survey. BMC Complementary Med Therap. 2023;23(1):392.

5

CHAPTER

Management of Nonfertility Signs and Symptoms

5.1 COSMETIC MEASURES

Urmila Nischal

INTRODUCTION

PCOS is associated with cosmetic concerns. The most common are acne, hair loss, hirsutism, and acanthosis nigricans. All these can cause significant psychological distress in the affected patients, whether adolescents, young adults or menopausal females. In fact, in most of them, these would be the signs that would make them seek help from dermatologists. Addressing these concerns is as important as treating the underlying hormonal issues. The dermatological manifestation can be a cause of significantly lower self-esteem. While treating these manifestations, it is important to understand that the therapy should be holistic, addressing the underlying pathology, suggesting lifestyle modifications and referring for cosmetic treatments.

5.1.1. What is the treatment for acne?

Draft recommendations:

5.1.1.1. For mild to moderate acne—IGA Grade 2-3: Combination of topical benzoyl peroxide either a face wash or cream/gel, along with topical retinoids like adapalene or tretinoin. *(High quality of evidence)*

5.1.1.2. For moderate to severe acne—IGA Grade 3-4 without hyperandrogenism:

Oral antibiotics like doxycycline/minocycline with the topical benzoyl peroxide and retinoids application.

For moderate to severe acne—i.e., IGA Grade 3-4 with diagnosed hyperandrogenism: Hormonal therapies with the newer generation oral contraceptive pills. If no response or suboptimal response add spironolactone. *(Moderate quality of evidence)*

5.1.1.3. For severe nodulocystic or resistant acne:

Oral isotretinoin with or without hormonal therapy. *(High quality of evidence)*

With topical agents like benzoyl peroxide/azelaic acid

5.1.1.4. All the grades can be supplemented by azelaic acid, salicylic acid gels/serums along with cosmetic procedures for better results. *(Clinical practice point)*

Summary of evidence: Acne is the most common skin disorder experienced by women! The causal relationship between acne and PCOS is well established.[1] Acne is a disorder of the pilosebaceous unit. The factors involved in the pathogenesis are (1) elevated sebum production, (2) increase in the pathogenic strain of *Cutibacterium acnes,* (3) Abnormal follicular keratinization, and (4) The innate immune response leads to the inflammatory component. The type and severity of the lesions manifested are further dependent on several internal and external factors like genetics, hormonal changes, diet, lifestyle, stress, and even environmental conditions.[2] All these factors need to be addressed while considering the treatment modalities for acne.

The grading of acne recommended by US FDA referred to as investigator global assessment (IGA) is as follows:[2]

Grade 0: Clear skin devoid of inflammatory or non-inflammatory lesions

Grade 1: "Almost clear", features rare noninflammatory lesions alongside no more than one small inflammatory lesion

Grade 2: Or "mild severity", includes some noninflammatory lesions with a few inflammatory lesions such as papules and pustules without any nodular lesions

Grade 3: Or "moderate severity", there are more noninflammatory and some inflammatory lesions, with no more than one nodular lesion

Grade 4: Severe, numerous noninflammatory, and inflammatory lesions, including a few nodular lesions.

Topical retinoids namely adapalene, tretinoin, tazarotene and trifarotene work on the RAR-β and RAR-γ receptors and improve follicular keratinization and reduce inflammatory lesions and comedones.[3] They form the mainstay of topical treatments. Trifarotene is the latest retinoid approved by the US FDA. Trifarotene due to its RAR-γ selectivity would be more effective with less adverse effects as compared to the other topical retinoids. Further studies are required to support this hypothesis. Topical benzoyl peroxide is the most commonly used antiacne agent with antimicrobial properties. It has anti-inflammatory and comedolytic properties. The advantage is that it prevents the development of antibiotic resistance to the topical antibiotics used. Available as a gel/cream or a wash. In patients not tolerating the gel/cream formulation, the face wash can be used with effective results.

Azelaic acid helps in reducing the erythema and the hyperpigmentation in acne patients. It has anti acne properties too. Available in gel and cream formulation it is quite well tolerated.

Salicylic acid, a beta-hydroxy acid, resolves mild acne due to its comedolytic, keratolytic, and mild anti-inflammatory properties while also having fungistatic and bacteriostatic properties.

Androgens play a major role in the pathogenesis of acne in PCOS. They increase the productions of the sebum, cause alteration in the composition of the lipids which incites the inflammatory reaction.[4]

Oral contraceptive pills reduce the gonadotropin release resulting in decreased androgen secretion from the ovaries.[4] They also have an anti-androgen effect on the sebaceous glands. The third generation progestins like desogestrel are preferred in view of their lowest androgenic activity.

Spironolactone is an antiandrogen (5α reductase inhibitor) which reduces sebum production and reduces acne.[4] Recommended dosage is 50–150 mg once a day after meals for better tolerability. It should always be given along with oral contraceptive pills as there is a risk of feminization of the male fetus. Spironolactone can be added when only oral contraceptive pills do not show the desired results after 3–6 cycles. Spironolactone needs to be continued for 6 months before reducing the dose.[4]

Long-term oral antibiotics should be avoided as there is a risk of antibiotic resistance and it also alters the gut microbiome which could worsen the acne.

Oral isotretinoin is most commonly prescribed medication by dermatologists for treating severe grades of acne. The advantage is that it works on all the factors involved in the pathogenesis of acne. The recommended starting dose is 0.3–0.5 mg/kg/day, up to a cumulative dose of 120–150 g.

Dermocosmetics are skin care actives that help in healing lesions, and improving the skin texture and pigmentation. They work synergistically with the pharmacological therapy.[5]

There are myriad of other factors such as stress, inadequate night sleep, cosmetics usage, unhealthy eating habits, smoking, and sedentary lifestyle which also play a significant role in acne and need to be addressed.[6]

Research gap: There is a paucity of clinical trials with topical treatments for acne in females with underlying PCOS. Also, there is a need to perform clinical studies of acne treatments in females both adolescents and adults with PCOS. There are no studies with recommendations for the duration of the therapies initiated.

5.1.2. What is the treatment for Hirsutism?

Draft recommendations:

5.1.2.1. For mild cases of hirsutism and patient-important hirsutism pharmacological therapy with OCPs alone as the first line of therapy. *(Moderate quality of evidence)*

5.1.2.2. For mild cases of hirsutism in patients who do not wish to conceive/have completed their family—Antiandrogens alone. *(Low quality of evidence)*

5.1.2.3. For moderate to severe cases of hirsutism—OCPs with antiandrogens. *(Moderate quality of evidence)*

5.1.2.4. For cases of patient-important hirsutism/mild cases where there is no response even after 6 months of monotherapy with OCPs add an antiandrogen alone. Continue the treatment for at least 6–9 months to label it as nonresponsive. *(Low quality of evidence)*

5.1.2.5. For hirsutism in females with high risk for venous thromboembolism—use a OCP with low dose ethinylestradiol and a low-risk progestin. *(Moderate quality of evidence)*

5.1.2.6. For all cases of hirsutism—laser hair reduction for dark hairs and electrolysis for gray hair is preferable to the temporary methods of hair removal alone. *(Low quality of evidence)*

5.1.2.7. One needs to offer holistic treatment including lifestyle changes to all patients of hirsutism irrespective of the severity of the hirsutism. Treatments should be designed taking into consideration the patient's needs and desires. *(Clinical practice point)*

Summary of evidence: Hirsutism is the presence of thick terminal hair in a male sexual pattern of distribution in females.[7] The modified Ferriman-Gallwey (mFG) scoring system is the gold standard for clinical grading of hirsutism.[8] The transition of the vellus hair to the terminal hair is androgen dependent. The severity of the hirsutism is not always correlated with the serum androgen levels. Therapeutic approach to treat hirsutism therefore involves 1) drug therapy targeting the action of androgens and 2. The hair removal methods.[8]

Combined oral contraceptive pills (OCPs) reduce the circulating androgens and are the first line of pharmacological therapy. They act by (a) suppressing Luteinizing hormone secretion which reduces the ovarian androgen production, (b) stimulate the hepatic production of SHBG which reduces the free circulating androgens, (c) reduces the adrenal androgen secretion slightly and also the binding of androgens to the receptors.[8]

Antiandrogens are added in cases of moderate to severe hirsutism and in cases where there is no response even after 6 months of treatment with OCPs.[8] In a placebo controlled trial with individual antiandrogens spironolactone 100 mg/d, finasteride 2.5–5 mg/d, and flutamide 500 mg/d, each showed a significant reduction in hirsutism scores. Due to the risk of hepatic toxicity spironolactone and finasteride are the preferred antiandrogens.

Temporary methods of hair removal such as shaving, plucking, waxing, threading, and applying depilatory creams are associated with side effects like allergies, pigmentation, rashes, ingrown hair, etc. These methods have to be repeated frequently and do not cause any reduction in the thickness or the number of hairs. The best modalities to address unwanted hair are laser hair reduction and electrolysis.

Electrolysis is recommended only for the gray hairs and not for the black hairs. Electrolysis is done by inserting an electric probe alongside the hair shaft into the skin and a current either direct, indirect or a blend of both, is delivered.[8] This heats the hair follicle thereby destroying it and preventing regrowth. This method is tedious and needs to target each hair follicle separately making it time-consuming. The results also depend on the skill of the treating physician. There is a risk of scarring, hyperpigmentation and hypopigmentation in some cases.

Lasers and light-based devices (intense pulse light) deliver permanent hair reduction. Lasers in skin work on the principle of selective photothermolysis. It means that a target or chromophore would absorb the light emitted in a particular wavelength depending on the properties of the target or the chromophore. In the case of laser hair reduction, the chromophore is melanin in the hair shafts.

The principle of the extended theory of photoablation is applied to laser photoablation. The melanin in the hair shaft absorbs the laser energy and transfers it to the surrounding follicular structures. This causes the destruction of the hair matrix and the hair bulge stem cells.

In the last decade lasers have become very popular because of the improved technologies and the skilled dermatologist. Different types of lasers available are Ruby laser (694 nm), Alexandrite laser (755 nm), Nd:YAG laser (1,064 nm), Diode laser (810 nm) and the latest addition is the Triple wavelength lasers.[9] Long pulsed Nd:YAG, diode and the triple wavelength lasers are best suited for the Indian skin types giving optimum results with minimum side effects.[10]

Laser session is repeated once in 4–6 weeks for facial hair and every 2–3 months for other body parts like the extremities.[11] An average of 6–8 sessions are required for a significant reduction. Patients with abnormal hormonal levels without medical treatment showed poor response to laser hair removal.

Intense pulse light (IPL) or broadband light (BBL) (500–1,200 nm) based lasers are less expensive than a true laser, IPL uses a flash lamp to fire high-intensity pulses of polychromatic, non-coherent light. Various filters can be used to narrow the wavelength of the light emitted. Not as effective as lasers.[11,12]

Topical 13.9% eflornithine cream is FDA-approved to reduce unwanted facial hair growth. Hair growth is significantly reduced by objective and subjective measures with twice-daily application for 8 weeks. The disadvantage is that it is not effective in 30% of cases and relapse to pretreatment status 8 weeks after discontinuation.

Research gap: There is paucity of data on the results of laser hair reduction for hirsutism patients with PCOS. The available trials for different therapies for hirsutism are constrained by lack of sample size, and blinded evaluation. We need more studies for our Indian patients as the skin type of Indian patients is different as compared to the Caucasian and the Asian population. The duration of the treatment to be continued for hirsutism is also not clear as most of the studies were conducted for a duration of 6–12 months.

5.1.3. What is the treatment for acanthosis nigricans?

Draft recommendations:

5.1.3.1. In cases of acanthosis nigricans with obesity—weight reduction, metformin, along with treatment of underlying PCOS. *(Low quality of evidence)*

5.1.3.2. In cases of acanthosis nigricans without obesity treatment should be directed to underlying PCOS. *(Low quality of evidence)*

5.1.3.3. Topical treatment can be added to all cases. Tretinoin 0.05–0.1% cream/gel application or calcipotriol 0.05%. *(Low quality of evidence)*

5.1.3.4. Cosmetic treatments are to be suggested as per the severity of the condition and the patient's requirements. *(Clinical practice point)*

Summary of evidence: Acanthosis nigricans is considered as a hallmark of insulin resistance. It is characterized by the presence of dark brown to black hyperpigmented velvety texture of the skin mainly in the neck, axillae, and knuckles. Also seen in the inframammary folds, cubital folds, and the groins.[13]

The incidence of acanthosis nigricans in females with PCOS varies with age, weight, pubertal status, severity of PCOS and presence of insulin resistance. The prevalence of acanthosis nigricans is 30–50% and it is noted to be up to 70–90% in obese females with PCOS.[13] Insulin resistance and hyperinsulinemia are the common mechanism that link acanthosis nigricans and PCOS.[14] Increased levels of insulin in hyperinsulinemia bind to the insulin-like growth factor-1 receptors and exert growth-promoting effects on the fibroblasts and keratinocytes, causing their proliferation, which is clinically manifested as dark thickened skin.[14] Therefore it is of utmost importance to target insulin resistance primarily in the treatment of acanthosis nigricans.

Insulin-sensitizing agents metformin and alpha-lipoic acid are recommended in acanthosis nigricans with obesity and insulin resistance.[14] They reduce insulin levels, improve insulin sensitivity and facilitate utilization of peripheral glucose, by preventing endocytosis of GLUT-4 receptor and by expression on the cell surface.[14]

Alpha-lipoic acid is a potent antioxidant and a naturally occurring cofactor of mitochondrial dehydrogenase complexes. It has been found to improve glucose metabolism in patients with type 2 diabetes.[14] Mechanism of action being direct engagement of the signaling pathways and consequent increased insulin sensitivity.

Dermatological treatments help in reducing the hyperpigmentation and thickness of the skin thereby improving the quality of life in these patients. Topical application of tretinoin 0.05–0.1% gel for 8 weeks is the most studied topical treatment. Topical vitamin D analogs like calcipotriol improves the thickness of the skin as it improves keratogenesis. They inhibit keratinocyte proliferation and promote differentiation by increasing keratinocyte intracellular calcium and cyclic GMP levels. Topical urea cream in a concentration of 10–20% and 10% salicylic cream are helpful with good tolerance. Other treatments are TCA and salicylic-mandelic peels which cause coagulation of the epidermal proteins, leading to collagen remodeling, improved keratinization, and decreased pigmentation.[15]

Interventions with lasers especially fractional CO_2 laser followed by retinoic peel have shown significant improvement in the lesions of acanthosis nigricans. Fractional CO_2 laser creates microcolumns of thermal damage surrounding normal skin, which helps in collagen induction and remodeling.[16] There is also a transepidermal elimination of the dermal contents, which helps in lightening the skin and significant improvement in the texture and thickness of the skin of the affected area.[16]

Research gap: The current literature is very limited with a small sample size and short follow-up time. No single treatment can be considered superior and definitive in giving results. There is a need for more targeted and definitive treatment modalities in acanthosis nigricans.

5.1.4. What is the treatment for female pattern hair loss?

Draft recommendation:

5.1.4.1. Topical minoxidil 5% application. *(High quality of evidence)*

5.1.4.2. Treatment of hyperandrogenemia with Spironolactone and oral combined contraceptive pills of third- and fourth-generation results in improvement. *(Moderate quality of evidence)*

5.1.4.3. Low-level of light therapy and PRP. *(Low quality of evidence)*

Summary of evidence: Female pattern hair loss (FPHL) is a distinct pattern of alopecia characterized by the conversion of the terminal hair follicles into vellus hair follicles and subsequent loss of the follicles. This results in thinning of the hair, widening of the partition and increased visibility of the scalp.[17] It may present in adolescence, early adulthood or in the peri/post-menopausal age group. The prevalence of FPHL in PCOS is about 20–30%, and only one-third of cases of FPHL have underlying hyperandrogenemia. The treatment aims at preventing the miniaturization of the hair follicles and sustaining the hair growth. Results are better if the treatment is started at the earliest as the miniaturization of the hairs is a progressive phenomenon.

Twice daily application of topical 5% minoxidil has robust evidence in the treatment of FPHL and hence it is the first line of management in the treatment of FPHL in cases of PCOS. The exact mechanism of action of topical minoxidil is not known. It prolongs the anagen phase and shortens the telogen phase, which is seen clinically as improved thickness of the hair and reduced hair shedding.[18] The results of topical minoxidil are variable as its action is dependent on the presence of sulfotransferase enzyme in the hair follicle, the levels of which vary in the population.

Oral antiandrogens: Most of the antiandrogens are not rigorously studied in FPHL. Results are better in cases with hyperandrogenism. While prescribing anti-androgens in women of childbearing age group counseling for contraception is important. Spironolactone in the dose of 50–200 mg per day for 6–12 months is the most common antiandrogen used in FPHL.[19] It competitively inhibits the androgen receptors in the target tissues, inhibits ovarian production of androgens, and reduces the levels of total testosterone. Bicalutamide is an antiandrogen which is used at low doses of 25–50 mg/day for treating FPHL who do not respond to spironolactone and combined oral contraceptive pills. Bicalutamide is a teratogenic agent and has side effects like transaminitis, peripheral edema and gastrointestinal complaints.[19] The combination of minoxidil with spironolactone is more effective than the combination of minoxidil and finasteride in women with FPHL.[18] 5-α reductase inhibitor finasteride is an off-label treatment for FPHL. Improvement was observed with a dose of 2.5–5 mg/day. Dutasteride another 5-α reductase inhibitor which binds both types I and II enzymes is three times more potent than finasteride in the inhibition of type II enzymes and 100 times more potent in the inhibition of type I enzymes. In a study, dutasteride was proposed to be more effective than finasteride in women <50 years of age. Dutasteride is classified as pregnancy category X because of teratogenicity and should have the same theoretical risk of breast cancer as mentioned in relation to finasteride.[18]

Oral contraceptive pills should be mandatory in the child-bearing group treated with antiandrogens. It is preferable to use 3rd (desogestrel and gestodene) or 4th (cyproterone acetate, chlormadinone acetate, and drospirenone) generation OCPs, which have less androgenic activity.

Low-level light therapy (LLLT) uses light in the wavelength of 600–1,100 nm to stimulate hair growth.[20] Being noninvasive it has become popular, it prolongs the anagen phase of hair growth, and prevents the premature conversion of anagen hairs into catagen hairs like minoxidil. LLLT may increase keratinocyte and fibroblast mitosis by generating reactive oxygen species (ROS) and antioxidants. LLLT decreases the inflammatory cytokines like prostaglandin E2 and increases the anti-inflammatory cytokines. The most commonly used devices have wavelengths in the range of 650–1,200 nm and fluences of 1–10 J/cm^2, with a power density of 3–90 mW/cm^2.[20] The treatment is usually for 15–20 min, three times a week for 6 months.

The alpha granules of the platelets are rich in platelet-derived growth factor (PDGF), vascular endothelial growth factor (VEGF), transforming growth factor beta (TGFβ), and insulin-like growth factors (IGF).[21] These growth factors promote angiogenesis and induction of stem cell differentiation, which result in a reduction in follicular apoptosis and promotion of follicular cell growth. The IGF-1-like growth factors negate the inhibitory effect of DHT on the hair follicles.

Combination therapies tend to give more promising results than monotherapies.[22] For results any form of therapy should be continued for a minimum of 6 months. A holistic approach with oral medications, topical applications and supportive in-clinic treatments yields satisfactory results.

Research gap: There is a lack of studies, which are pertaining to FPHL with PCOS. The sample size is small and most of the studies do not have randomized controls. High-quality randomized control trials are required to standardize the treatment protocols in this population.

5.1.5. How effective are cosmetic procedures?

Draft recommendation:

5.1.5.1. Cosmetic procedures like lasers, chemical peels, PRP are additive and do work synergistically with medical therapy and are effective in reducing dermatological manifestations. *(Moderate quality of evidence)*

Summary of evidence: Lasers for hair reduction are very well-studied. And thanks to the availability of newer and improved technologies, it is one of the most commonly performed treatments in a dermatologist's office. The safety of lasers has been proved in darker Indian skin types as well.[23]

Chemical peels consist of different organic acids like salicylic acid, glycolic acid, mandelic acid, jasmonic acid, trichloroacetic acid in different strengths and combinations, which results in exfoliation of the superficial layers of the skin, resulting in improved texture and color of the skin.[24] They also help in neocollagenesis and thus in improvement of the scars, fine lines and wrinkles.[24]

Various randomized controlled trials have supported the efficacy of PRP in the treatment of FPHL. Though there is a lack of standardization, PRP therapy is a useful adjunctive tool in the treatment of FPHL.[25]

Research gap: Double blind randomized controlled trials targeting specific demographic population is required to further guide the clinical practice and generate evidence. There is a need to standardize the various cosmetic treatments.

CONCLUSION

PCOS is associated with dermatological manifestations like acne, hirsutism, FPHL, hyperpigmentation, and acanthosis nigricans, which cause social embarrassment, low self-esteem and psychological distress. Improving these imperfections is very rewarding for the patients. The aim of PCOS treatment should be to provide holistic management targeting the underlying hormonal imbalance and the external signs. Cosmetic procedures are minimally invasive treatments with very little or no downtime. They include chemical peels, lasers for collagen remodeling (resurfacing lasers), and lasers for hair removal. The thick terminal hair in hirsutism that cannot be resolved only by medical therapy can be reduced with laser therapy. Chemical peels are an effective treatment for acne and associated pigmentation. These treatments work synergistically with the medical therapy. Resurfacing lasers like fractional CO_2 lasers help in treating active acne as well as atrophic scars, which cause significant disfigurement in female patients. Early initiation of the treatments is prudent to prevent further deterioration of the signs like FPHL. Treatments should be designed taking into account the patient's needs and desires too!

REFERENCES

1. Ramezani Tehrani F, Behboudi-Gandevani S, Bidhendi Yarandi R, et al. Prevalence of acne vulgaris among women with polycystic ovary syndrome: a systemic review and meta-analysis. Gynecol Endocrinol. 2021;37:392-405.
2. Neill AM, Gallo RL. Host-microbiome interactions and recent progress into understanding the biology of acne vulgaris. Microbiome. 2018;6:177.
3. Baldwin H, Webster G, Stein Gold L, et al. 50 Years of topical retinoids for acne: evolution of treatment. Am J Clin Dermatol. 2021;22:315-27.
4. Carmina E, Dreno B, Lucky WA, et al. Female Adult Acne and Androgen Excess: A Report From the Multidisciplinary Androgen Excess and PCOS Committee. J Endocr Soc. 2022;6(3):bvac003.
5. Dreno B, Araviiskaia E, Berardesca E, et al. The science of dermocosmetics and its role in dermatology. J Eur Acad Dermatol Venereol. 2014;28:1409-11.
6. Poli F, Auffret N, Claudel JP, et al. AFAST: an adult female acne treatment algorithm for daily clinical practice. Eur J Dermatol. 2018;28(1):101-3.
7. Barrionuevo P, Nabhan M, Altayar O, et al. Treatment options for hirsutism: a systematic review and network meta-analysis. J Clin Endocrinol Metab. 2018;103(4):1258-64.
8. Martin KA, Anderson RR, Chang RJ, et al. Evaluation and Treatment of Hirsutism in Premenopausal Women: An Endocrine Society Clinical Practice Guideline. J Clin Endocrinol Metab. 2018;103(4):1233-57.
9. Lee CM. Laser-assisted hair removal for facial hirsutism in women: a review of evidence. J Cosmet Laser Ther. 2018;20(3):140-4.
10. Raj Kirit EP, Sivuni A, Ponugupati S, et al. Efficacy and safety of triple wavelength laser hair reduction in skin types IV to V. J Cosmet Dermatol. 2021;20(4):1117-23.
11. Rafi S, Budania A, Bhardwaj A, et al. Efficacy and safety of diode laser for facial hair reduction in hirsutism-a clinico-trichoscopic evaluation. J Cutan Aesthet Surg. 2024;17(1):19-24.
12. Tan K, Coster T, Mousa A, et al. Laser and light-based therapies for hirsutism management in women with polycystic ovarian syndrome: a systematic review. JAMA Dermatol. 2024;160(7):746-57.
13. Das A, Datta D, Kassir M, et al. Acanthosis nigricans: a review. J Cosmet Dermatol. 2020;19:1857-65.
14. Sharma YK, Chauhan S, Singh P, et al. Correlation of cutaneous manifestations with body mass index, blood glucose, and hormonal levels in patients with polycystic ovarian disease. Indian Dermatol. Online J. 2020;11:378-81.

15. Treesirichod A, Thaneerat N, Kangvanskol W. A comparison of the efficacy and safety profiles of 10% salicylic acid and 10% urea creams in treating acanthosis nigricans in adolescents: a randomized double-blinded study. Arch Dermatol Res. 2023;315(7):2091-7.
16. Abu Oun AA, Ahmed NA, Hafiz HSA. Comparative study between fractional carbon dioxide laser versus retinoic acid chemical peel in the treatment of acanthosis nigricans. J Cosmet Dermatol. 2022;21:1023-30.
17. Khera R, Pandey A, Chandar AK, et al. Effects of weight-loss medications on cardiometabolic risk profiles: a systematic review and network meta-analysis. Gastroenterology. 2018;154(5):1309-19.e7.
18. Sadeghzadeh Bazargan A, Tavana Z, Dehghani A, et al. The efficacy of the combination of topical minoxidil and oral spironolactone compared with the combination of topical minoxidil and oral finasteride in women with androgenic alopecia, female and male hair loss patterns: a blinded randomized clinical trial. J Cosmet Dermatol. 2024;23:543-51.
19. Jha AK, Zeeshan MD, Singh A, et al. Efficacy and safety of spironolactone versus bicalutamide in female pattern hair loss: a retrospective comparative study. Australas J Dermatol. 2024;65:437-43.
20. Kaiser MA, Almeida SM, Rodriguez M, et al. Low-level light therapy and minoxidil combination treatment in androgenetic alopecia: a review of the literature. Skin Appendage Disord. 2023;9(2):1-7.
21. Tawfik AA, Osman MAR. The effect of autologous activated platelet-rich plasma injection on female pattern hair loss: a randomized placebo-controlled study. J Cosmet Dermatol. 2018;17:47-53.
22. Zhou Y, Chen C, Qu Q, et al. The effectiveness of combination therapies for androgenetic alopecia: a systematic review and meta-analysis. Dermatol Ther. 2020;33(4):e13741.
23. Kao YC, Lin DZ, Kang YN, et al. Efficacy of laser in hair removal: a network meta-analysis. J Cosmet Laser Ther. 2023;25(1-4):7-19.
24. Tam C, Khong J, Tam K, et al. A comprehensive review of non-energy-based treatments for atrophic acne scarring. Clin Cosmet Investig Dermatol. 2022;15:455-69.
25. Torabi P, Behrangi E, Goodarzi A, et al. A systematic review of the effect of platelet-rich plasma on androgenetic alopecia of women. Dermatol Ther. 2020;33(6):e13835.

5.2 PHARMACOTHERAPY

Rakhi Singh

INTRODUCTION

In PCOS lifestyle management is the first line of management followed by the use of pharmacological agents like combined oral contraceptive pills (COCP), insulin sensitizers (metformin, inositol, and GLP-1 agonist) and antiandrogens (cyproterone acetate, spironolactone, flutamide, and finasteride). Pharmacotherapy is usually directed to the key symptoms that are of concern to women with PCOS and thus should be individualized.

COCP is commonly prescribed for cycle irregularity and clinical hyperandrogenism. Antiandrogenic pills are more effective in controlling hirsutism and androgenic symptoms. Insulin resistance is seen in both lean and obese PCOS. Insulin sensitizers are commonly used in adjunct with COCPs, in obese, overweight women to improve weight loss and metabolic parameters. Though pharmacotherapy in PCOS is evidence-based but usually off-label and therefore counseling by the clinician about the benefits and side effects is essential.

5.2.1. What is the role of combined oral contraceptives (COCP)?

Draft recommendation:

5.2.1.1. The combined oral contraceptive pill (COCP) is recommended in reproductive-age women with PCOS for the management of hirsutism and/or irregular menstrual cycles. *(Moderate quality of evidence)*

5.2.1.2. The COCP could be used in adolescents at risk or with a clear diagnosis of PCOS for management of hirsutism and/or irregular menstrual cycles. *(Moderate quality of evidence)*

5.2.1.3. Low dose of ethinylestradiol (<30 µg) in the COCP is preferred for treating hirsutism. *(Moderate quality of evidence)*

5.2.1.4. The 35 µg ethinylestradiol with cyproterone acetate should be used only as second-line therapy over other COCPs, as it is associated with adverse effects, including venous thromboembolic risks. *(Moderate quality of evidence)*

5.2.1.5. Progestin-only oral contraceptives may be considered for endometrial protection, though the evidence in women with PCOS is limited. *(Low quality of evidence)*

Summary of evidence: When prescribing COCPs in adults, adolescent PCOS, and adolescents at risk of PCOS natural estrogen preparations and the lowest effective estrogen doses of 20–30 µg of ethinylestradiol or equivalent should be used. Before COCP is initiated one needs to rule out all contraindications. COCP play a crucial role in managing PCOS, particularly in addressing menstrual irregularities, and hyperandrogenism and providing endometrial protection. The COCP can improve symptoms through multiple pathways including:

- Direct inhibition of ovarian androgen production
- Increased hepatic production of sex hormone binding globulin (SHBG), which reduces free androgen availability
- Direct antiandrogenic effects of newer progestins

COCPs are highly effective in regulating menstrual cycles, leading to more regular, less painful, and lighter periods. Their use also reduces abnormal uterine bleeding (AUB), premenstrual syndrome (PMS) symptoms, and lowers the risk of ovarian and endometrial cancers caused by prolonged unopposed estrogen exposure.[1] They help decrease hyperandrogenism by raising levels of sex hormone-binding globulin (SHBG). COCPs are also effective in managing symptoms of androgen excess, such as hirsutism and alopecia. When COCP is combined with lifestyle modification and metformin it provides an additional benefit. The use of COCP has shown improvement on multiple aspects of quality of life (QoL), although the evidence supporting this is of very low certainty. Additionally, weight, testosterone, and insulin levels tend to be lower after COCP treatment.[2]

Research gaps: COCP is an off-label treatment for PCOS without classical clinical features. Research is needed to understand how different formulations of COCPs affect individuals differently based on their genetic makeup, severity of PCOS symptoms, and other coexisting health conditions, to optimize treatment plans. Before starting COCP in women with PCOS, one needs to counsel each of them on the benefits and risks of using COCP. More research is needed to assess the prolonged use of COCPs in PCOS and their impact on metabolic health.

5.2.2. Which is the most effective and safest COCP available and how long should they be continued?

Draft recommendation:

5.2.2.1. Estrogen-containing COCP is effective and recommended in the treatment of inflammatory acne in females. *(High quality of evidence)*

5.2.2.2. Both ethinylestradiol/drospirenone and ethinylestradiol/cyproterone acetate combinations improve hyperandrogenic parameters significantly without affecting the insulin resistance adversely in Indian women with PCOS. *(High quality of evidence)*

5.2.2.3. Progestin-only oral contraceptives may be considered for endometrial protection. *(Moderate quality of evidence)*

5.2.2.4. Use of lowest effective dose of 20–30 μg of ethinylestradiol or equivalent is effective and safe. *(Clinical practice points)*

5.2.2.5. COCPs could be given for 3–6 months for cycle regulation. *(Clinical practice points)*

5.2.2.6. COCPs could be given for 6 months for a reduction in hirsutism and acne. *(Clinical practice points)*

5.2.2.7. OCPs need to be stopped in the presence of any side effects or if abnormal glucose tolerance or dyslipidemia is detected. *(Low quality of evidence)*

5.2.2.8. After initial evaluation with all contraindications ruled out COCPs can be given for longer periods and regular follow-up advised. *(Clinical practice points)*

Summary of evidence: A systematic review indicates that COCPs containing cyproterone acetate (CPA) are most effective for managing hirsutism and acne, but they carry an increased risk of venous thromboembolism (VTE) due to the high content of ethinylestradiol (EE) and CPA. Using cyproterone acetate in combination with a lower dose of EE or natural estrogens may be a promising option for the future.[2] The progestins identified in the included studies were:[1]

First generation: Chlormadinone acetate (CMA)

Second generation: Levonorgestrel (LNG)

Third generation: Desogestrel (DSG) and gestodene

Fourth generation: Drospirenone (DRSP) and dienogest (DNG)

Others: Cyproterone acetate (CPA)

Among the available oral contraceptives, those with lower doses of ethinylestradiol are preferred, as higher doses do not offer additional benefits in managing hyperandrogenism symptoms. Higher doses of ethinylestradiol are associated with an increased risk of venous thrombosis. All COCPs are considered equally effective in women with PCOS.[2,3] Progestin-only oral contraceptives may be considered for endometrial protection, as women with PCOS, who often experience chronic anovulation, are at an increased risk of developing endometrial carcinoma due to unopposed estrogen action. A follow-up visit is recommended three months after starting COCP therapy to monitor for any potential side effects, such as hypertension or thrombosis.

The optimal duration of COCP therapy has not been clearly defined in current guidelines. However, after six months of treatment, most women with hirsutism show clinical improvement. Once weight loss is achieved, it may be advisable to discontinue COCPs due to their potential adverse effects on the metabolic profile. It is recommended to reassess the patient after six months, and future therapy should be determined by weighing the risks against the benefits.[1] The risk of hypertension increases by 13% for every five years of COCP use. Long-term concerns associated with prolonged COCP use include an elevated risk of thrombosis, deep vein thrombosis (DVT), venous thromboembolism (VTE), cardiovascular issues, and cancer. These risks are further heightened in individuals with high BMI, obesity, and dyslipidemia.[4]

Research gaps: Comparative studies on the different generations and types of progestins are needed to guide clinical decisions. More research is needed on COCP effects regarding long-term metabolic health, bone density, and mental health outcomes. Research is also needed to determine the ideal length of treatment that balances efficacy in symptom management with minimizing long-term risks, particularly for conditions like hirsutism. Studies could explore the outcomes of different discontinuation strategies and their impact on long-term health.

5.2.3. What precautions one needs to take when prescribing COCP in adolescents and adults?

Draft recommendation:

5.2.3.1. While prescribing COCPs to women with PCOS, the relative and absolute contraindications and side effects of COCPs need to be considered. *(Clinical practice point)*

5.2.3.2. COCPs chosen should not worsen the metabolic profile of the woman with PCOS. *(Clinical practice point)*

Summary of evidence: Before prescribing COCPs for any indication, clinicians should routinely assess each patient on an individual basis, taking into account the presence of relative risk factors such as age, smoking, obesity, diabetes, dyslipidemia, and any personal or family history of venous thromboembolic events or thrombophilia. Some absolute contraindications to COCP use include thromboembolic disorder, cerebrovascular or coronary artery disease, uncontrolled hypertension, known thrombogenic mutations, stroke, breast cancer, undiagnosed abnormal genital bleeding, benign or malignant liver tumors, jaundice with previous OCP use and Hypersensitivity to OCPs.[1]

Other points to consider apart from contraindications and drug interactions are:[5]

- COCPs with 35 μg EE and cyproterone acetate should not be used as first-line due to the higher risk for venous thrombosis.
- Estrogen in COCP may affect the peak bone mass during adolescent age (<14 years) and young adults. If the need arises for the use of COCP in adolescents, then the preferred drugs like Drospirenone should be used.[6]

The benefits of using the COCPs in women with PCOS should outweigh the risks of the treatment.

Research gaps: More studies are needed to refine risk stratification models, particularly in diverse populations with varying genetic backgrounds and health conditions.

5.2.4. What is the role of Insulin sensitizers (metformin and myoinositols) and should all women with PCOS be given insulin sensitizers?

Draft recommendations:

5.2.4.1. Metformin offers greater benefits in high metabolic risk groups including those with diabetes risk factors, and impaired glucose tolerance. *(Clinical practice point)*

5.2.4.2. Metformin alone should be considered in adults with PCOS and a BMI ≥25 kg/m^2 for anthropometric and metabolic outcomes including insulin resistance, glucose, and lipid profiles. *(Very low quality of evidence)*

5.2.4.3. Could be given to adolescents with BMI ≥25 kg/m^2 for the management of weight and metabolic outcomes if LSM is not effective. *(Very low quality of evidence)*

5.2.4.4. Where COCP is contraindicated, not accepted or not tolerated, metformin may be considered for irregular menstrual cycles. *(Clinical practice point)*

5.2.4.5. Myoinositol, part of the vitamin B complex, could be considered for women with PCOS, noting limited harm, and potential for improvement in metabolic measures. *(Very low quality of evidence)*

5.2.4.6. Metformin + myoinositol combination treatment in obese patients with PCOS has demonstrated better improvement in hormonal and metabolic parameters compared to metformin or myoinositol alone. *(Clinical practice point)*

5.2.4.7. Metformin is to be considered over inositol in hirsutism and central obesity. *(Very low quality of evidence)*

5.2.4.8. First-line therapy which should be recommended to all women with PCOS is lifestyle intervention (behavior, diet, and physical activity). *(Very low quality of evidence)*

5.2.4.9. Insulin sensitizers should be given in women with BMI >25 and/or those who have glucose intolerance. *(Very low quality of evidence)*

5.2.4.10. Insulin sensitizers which include metformin and inositols are indicated when lifestyle intervention is not effective. *(Clinical practice point)*

Summary of evidence: A key pathophysiological feature of PCOS is insulin resistance, characterized by decreased insulin action, which leads to disturbances in fatty acid metabolism, hyperandrogenism, and an exacerbation of PCOS symptoms. Insulin resistance is observed in 75% of lean women and 95% of women with a higher BMI, as documented by clamp studies.[4,7]

Metformin, a low-cost and widely available medication, has been used extensively as an insulin sensitizer for over seventy years in type 2 diabetes and for several decades in PCOS management. Inositols, on the other hand, are considered weak insulin sensitizers.

Insulin sensitizers are beneficial in reducing HOMA-IR, fasting glucose levels, and improving lipid profiles. They also help regulate menstrual cycles, which can enhance reproductive outcomes when used for six months or longer. Meta-analysis indicates that metformin is more effective than placebo in reducing BMI, waist-to-hip ratio (WHR), testosterone levels, fasting glucose, total cholesterol, triglycerides, C-reactive protein (CRP), and HOMA-IR.[7]

Metformin, in combination with inositol, significantly improves HOMA-IR, leading to regular menstrual cycles and increased live birth rates.

Metformin is preferred over inositol in cases of central obesity, hirsutism, and other hyperandrogenic symptoms. The combination of metformin and inositol enhances ovarian function, reduces elevated luteinizing hormone levels, and lowers hyperandrogenism by decreasing both total and free testosterone levels while increasing sex hormone-binding globulin (SHBG).[8] Therapy with myoinositols may be more expensive than metformin; however, it generally has fewer side effects.

Insulin sensitizers are not recommended for all women with PCOS, despite the fact that up to 90% of women with PCOS experience insulin resistance. Lifestyle interventions, including a calorie-restricted diet, regular exercise, and behavioral modifications, are the first-line treatment for all women with PCOS. When implemented effectively, these lifestyle changes can lead to weight loss and improvements in both metabolic and hormonal parameters.[7,9]

Research gaps: While metformin is shown to be effective in improving various metabolic and reproductive outcomes in PCOS, more research is needed on its long-term safety and efficacy. Myoinositol is suggested to have limited harm and potential benefits for improving metabolic measures in PCOS. Further research is needed to fully understand its efficacy as a standalone treatment. There is insufficient evidence regarding the types, dosages, or combinations of inositol for adults and adolescents with PCOS.

Research should explore how individualized treatment plans that combine lifestyle interventions and insulin sensitizers can be optimized based on factors such as BMI, glucose tolerance, and individual response to therapy.

5.2.5. How long to continue Insulin sensitizers in adolescents and adults?

Draft recommendation:

5.2.5.1. Insulin sensitizers should be continued in the presence of impaired glucose tolerance and type 2 diabetes mellitus. *(High quality of evidence)*

5.2.5.2. Could be used for more than 6 months in woman without impaired glucose tolerance or type 2 diabetes with regular follow ups, for better and sustained weight loss. *(Clinical practice point)*

5.2.5.3. Insulin sensitizers could be given as an adjunct to lifestyle intervention for a duration of 6 months. *(Clinical practice point)*

Summary of evidence: The exact duration of metformin therapy is not discussed in any guidelines. In clinical settings, insulin sensitizers should be given till the desired weight loss is achieved, till the abnormal glucose parameters return to normal, with regular follow ups. Studies with long term use of metformin (>1 year) in PCOS indicate better and sustained weight loss and less conversion to glucose intolerance in these women.[10] Nevertheless the clinicians should be aware of the side effects of long term use of metformin, which includes peripheral neuropathy, vitamin B12 deficiency.[8,11]

Research gaps: While insulin sensitizers are typically used for 6 months or more, there is a need for research to determine the optimal duration and dosage of treatment for maximizing benefits and minimizing side effects in PCOS management.

5.2.6. Is combination therapy of COCP and metformin more beneficial?

Draft recommendations:

5.2.6.1. COCP therapy has benefits for management of hyperandrogenism and menstrual regulation and metformin has beneficial effects on metabolic profile. *(Clinical practice point)*

5.2.6.2. Metformin and COCP combination could work better in adults with PCOS with a BMI > 30 kg/m^2, diabetes risk factors, impaired glucose tolerance or high-risk ethnic groups. *(Clinical practice point)*

5.2.6.3. Combination of COCPs and metformin could be recommended in adults and adolescents with obesity/metabolic complications when lifestyle modification (LSM) and COCP is not effective. *(Clinical practice point)*

Summary of evidence: Although combining metformin with COCP provides additional benefits, these do not exceed the advantages of COCP combined with lifestyle interventions. Therefore, this combination should be considered when COCP and lifestyle changes alone have not achieved the desired outcomes. It is also important to note that this combination may lead to more mild gastrointestinal side effects, which could affect adherence. Women with PCOS who have a higher BMI may experience the most significant benefits from adding metformin to COCP therapy.[11]

Research gaps: Further studies are needed to assess the long-term effects of combining metformin with COCP on metabolic health, reproductive outcomes, and overall quality of life. Research should focus on determining the optimal dosage and duration of metformin when used in combination with COCP.

5.2.7. What is the role of antiandrogens and which group of women benefit from antiandrogen therapy?

Draft recommendation:

5.2.7.1. Antiandrogens are effective in treating hirsutism. *(Very low quality of evidence)*

5.2.7.2. Antiandrogens with COCPs could be tried for managing alopecia. *(Low quality of evidence)*

5.2.7.3. Women on antiandrogen therapy should avoid pregnancy. *(Clinical practice point)*

5.2.7.4. Antiandrogens could be given to manage hirsutism, where 6 months of COCP and/or cosmetic therapy is not effective. *(Very low quality of evidence)*

5.2.7.5. Antiandrogens could be given to treat hirsutism in women in whom COCP are either contraindicated or not tolerated. *(Clinical practice point)*

Summary of evidence: Antiandrogens are a class of medications that lower circulating androgen levels and are commonly used to alleviate symptoms related to hyperandrogenism. Since hyperandrogenemia is a significant issue in PCOS, antiandrogens can be effective in managing troublesome symptoms such as hirsutism and alopecia. Several antiandrogens are available for treating hirsutism in PCOS, including finasteride, flutamide, bicalutamide, spironolactone, and cyproterone acetate (CPA).[12]

For women with PCOS primarily concerned about hirsutism, it is recommended to start treatment with COCPs combined with lifestyle interventions for six months. If these approaches are ineffective or if the condition significantly impacts the woman's psychological well-being, anti-androgens may be considered. Additionally, for women with PCOS who have metabolic issues such as dyslipidemia, glucose intolerance, or hypertension, or who cannot use COCPs due to contraindications, antiandrogens can be recommended for managing hirsutism alongside local cosmetic hair removal treatments.[13]

Research gap: Research is needed to compare the effectiveness and safety of various anti-androgens (such as finasteride, flutamide, bicalutamide, spironolactone, and CPA) in treating hirsutism and alopecia in women with PCOS and their effect on the metabolic profile. More detailed studies are warranted with larger number of participants to determine the beneficial effects of antiandrogens.

5.2.8. Should antiandrogens be used in combination with other drugs to be more effective?

Draft recommendation:

5.2.8.1. Antiandrogens can be used to treat hirsutism with effective contraception if there is suboptimal response with 6 months of treatment with COCP and or cosmetic therapy or where there is a contraindication for use of COCP or when COCPs are poorly tolerated. *(Very low quality of evidence)*

5.2.8.2. Antiandrogens with COCPs could be tried for managing alopecia and to correct menstrual irregularity. *(Very low quality of evidence)*

5.2.8.3. In case there is pregnancy when antiandrogens are used there is a risk of incomplete development of external genital structures of male fetuses. *(Clinical practice point)*

Summary of evidence: Antiandrogens used with COCPs are definitely more effective in management of hirsutism and alopecia.[13] Additional contraception should be advised to women on antiandrogen therapy, as these drugs can have deleterious effects on the growing fetus. While giving in combination therapy, side effect profile should be kept in mind.

Antiandrogens, prescribed include:

- Spironolactone at 25–100 mg/day appears to have lower risks of adverse effects
- Cyproterone acetate at doses of ≥10 mg is not advised due to an increased risk of developing meningioma
- Finasteride has an increased risk of liver toxicity
- Flutamide and bicalutamide have an increased risk of severe liver toxicity Best evidence is seen for spironolactone.

Research gaps: There is limited evidence on use of antiandrogens in PCOS in view of small numbers of studies and limited numbers of participants. There is a gap in understanding how best to combine antiandrogens with other treatments like COCPs, insulin sensitizers, and local cosmetic hair removal therapies for optimal management of hirsutism.

CONCLUSION

PCOS is a common endocrine disorder that is associated with diverse symptoms and features, and an increased risk of long-term sequelae which include type 2 diabetes and cardiovascular disease. Pharmacotherapy for PCOS should be directed at the key symptoms of the individual patient. The COCP or metformin may be prescribed for irregular periods. COCP is preferred over antiandrogens for the treatment of hirsutism and acne. Metformin is beneficial for reducing excess body weight and improving hormonal and metabolic abnormalities, especially in women with a BMI of >25 kg/m^2. Inositol appears to have limited benefits for metabolic outcomes, but is associated with fewer gastrointestinal side effects as compared to metformin and therefore can be used in those women who cannot tolerate metformin. Lifestyle modification is an important and first-line treatment in women with PCOS along with pharmacotherapy. Anti-obesity drugs may be considered for weight management in addition to lifestyle interventions.

KEYPOINTS

1. *Combined oral contraceptive pills:* These are most commonly prescribed to manage PCOS symptoms like irregular periods, acne, and hirsutism.

They work by regulating menstrual cycles and reducing androgens which can help with acne and hair growth.

2. *Metformin:* Primarily used to manage insulin resistance, a common feature of PCOS. Metformin helps improve insulin sensitivity, which can regulate menstrual cycles and support weight management. It may also aid in lowering testosterone levels.
3. *Inositols:* These are often used as supplements to improve insulin sensitivity and ovarian function. The most commonly used forms are myoinositol and D-chiro-inositol. They can help in restoring normal menstrual cycles and improving ovarian function.
4. *Antiandrogen therapy:* Medications such as spironolactone are used to counteract the effects of excess androgens (male hormones) in PCOS. This therapy helps manage symptoms like acne, hirsutism, and hair thinning by blocking androgen receptors.

Each treatment has specific benefits and is often chosen based on individual symptoms and health goals.

REFERENCES

1. Forslund M, Melin J, Alesi S, et al. Combined oral contraceptive pill compared with no medical treatment in the management of polycystic ovary syndrome: a systematic review. Clin Endocrinol (Oxf). 2023;99(1):79-91.
2. Forslund M, Melin J, Alesi S, et al. Different kinds of oral contraceptive pills in polycystic ovary syndrome: a systematic review and meta-analysis. Eur J Endocrinol. 2023;189(1):S1-S16.
3. Akre S, Sharma K, Chakole S, et al. Recent advances in the management of polycystic ovary syndrome: a review article. Cureus. 2022;14(8):e27689.
4. Teede H, Tassone EC, Piltonen T, et al. Effect of the combined oral contraceptive pill and/or metformin in the management of polycystic ovary syndrome: a systematic review with meta-analyses. Clin Endocrinol (Oxf). 2019;91:479-89.
5. Morgante G, Cappelli V, Troìa L, et al. Evaluation of different antiandrogenic progestins on clinical and biochemical variables in polycystic ovary syndrome. Eur J Contracept Reprod Health Care. 2020;25(3):176-81.
6. Witchel SF, Oberfield SE, Peña AS. Polycystic ovary syndrome: pathophysiology, presentation, and treatment with emphasis on adolescent girls. J Endocr Soc. 2019;3(8):1545-73.
7. Joham AE, Norman RJ, Stener-Victorin E, et al. Polycystic ovary syndrome. Lancet Diabetes Endocrinol. 2022;10(9):668-80. Erratum in: Lancet Diabetes Endocrinol. 2022;10(11):e11.
8. Unfer V, Facchinetti F, Orrù B, et al. Myo-inositol effects in women with PCOS: a meta-analysis of randomized controlled trials. Endocr Connect. 2017;6(8):647-58.
9. Melin J, Forslund M, Alesi S, et al. Response to Letter to the Editor from de Zegher and Ibáñez: 'Metformin and combined oral contraceptive pills in the management of polycystic ovary syndrome: a systematic review and meta-analysis. J Clin Endocrinol Metab. 2024.

10. Jensterle M, Kravos NA, Ferjan S, et al. Long-term efficacy of metformin in overweight-obese PCOS: longitudinal follow-up of retrospective cohort. Endocr Connect. 2020;9(1):44-54.
11. Fraison E, Kostova E, Moran LJ, et al. Metformin versus the combined oral contraceptive pill for hirsutism, acne, and menstrual pattern in polycystic ovary syndrome. Cochrane Database Syst Rev. 2020;8(8):CD005552.
12. Alesi S, Forslund M, Melin J, et al. Efficacy and safety of anti-androgens in the management of polycystic ovary syndrome: a systematic review and meta-analysis of randomised controlled trials. EClinicalMedicine. 2023;63:102162.
13. Rajashekar S, Giri Ravindran S, Kakarla M, et al. Spironolactone versus oral contraceptive pills in the treatment of adolescent polycystic ovarian syndrome: a systematic review. Cureus. 2022;14(5):e25340.

5.3 ROLE OF ANTIOBESITY DRUGS IN ADOLESCENTS AND ADULT WOMEN WITH PCOS

Pratik Tambe

INTRODUCTION

Obesity is a significant public health concern due to its association with various health problems, including diabetes, heart disease and certain types of cancer **(Flowchart 1)**. Obesity has now been identified as a key component of the "global syndemic", a condition which is exemplified by obesity, under-/malnutrition and climate change as the most important modern health issues faced worldwide by civilization and the environment, especially in the years to come.[1]

Antiobesity medications (AOMs) are indicated when body mass index (BMI) is ≥30 kg/m^2 or ≥27 kg/m^2 with obesity-related comorbidity. It is also advocated if lifestyle modification attempts have failed in reducing

Flowchart 1: Obesity associated morbidities.

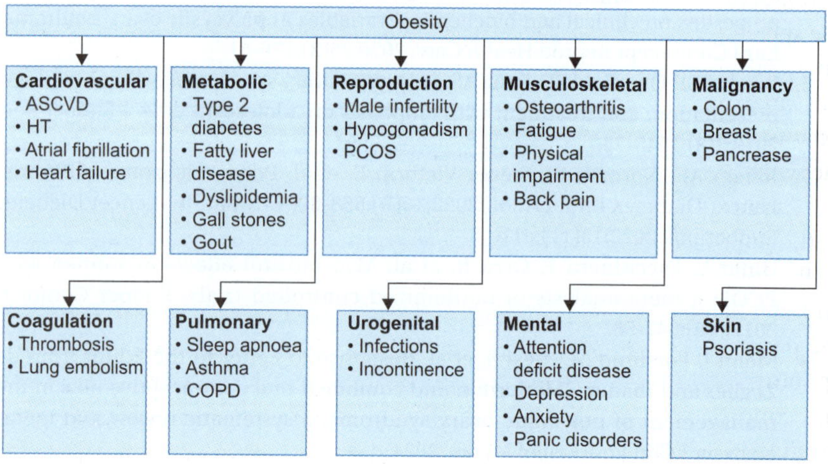

obesity. Antiobesity medication can be used in combination with lifestyle modification. Current antiobesity drugs act through several potential mechanisms, including increasing energy expenditure, suppressing appetite, inhibiting digestive enzymes, or interfering with the absorption of fat or sugar from food at the intestinal tract level.

5.3.1. What are antiobesity drugs used for weight reduction and which of them are available in India?

Draft recommendation:

5.3.1.1. Orlistat, phentermine/topiramate, naltrexone/bupropion, glucagon-like peptide-1 (GLP-1) receptor agonists-liraglutide, and semaglutide are approved for nonsyndromic obesity. Tirzepatide and incretins are currently being investigated in different phases of clinical trials. *(Low quality of evidence)*

5.3.1.2. Orlistat, liraglutide, semaglutide, and tirzepatide are the drugs available in India apart from the ayurvedic drugs used for weight loss. *(Clinical practice point)*

5.3.1.3. Antiobesity medications like glucagon-like peptide-1 (GLP-1) receptor (liraglutide and semaglutide), and orlistat, could be used in addition to active lifestyle interventions, for the management of obese PCOS. *(Very low quality of evidence)*

5.3.1.4. Combining medications with complementary mechanisms of action could be a management strategy in those who are unable to maintain weight loss or have further weight loss after reaching a weight loss plateau. *(Low quality of evidence)*

Summary of evidence: Antiobesity drugs act centrally, to reduce appetite and increase satiety, and secondarily, in the gastrointestinal tract to slow gastric emptying. These medications are capable of improving weight loss and metabolic parameters, with variable potency and effects depending on the specific drug that has been used.[2] The currently available AOMs result in about 10% weight loss with a dose that is tolerable without side effects.[3] Even this small amount of weight loss improves the severity of comorbidities that exist with obesity. It is important to monitor patients on AOMs for abuse, tachyphylaxis, and other adverse effects.

The mechanism of action of GLP1 agonist is multifactorial, with actions in the gut (decreased Gastric emptying and gastrointestinal motility), brain (↓ food intake, reward behavior, and palatability), liver (↓ gluconeogenesis and steatosis), muscle (↑ insulin sensitivity and glucose uptake) and in the pancreas (↑ insulin secretion and synthesis ↓ glucagon secretion and apoptosis and ↑ β-cell survival). This in turn improves the metabolic function and contributes to weight loss.[3] Liraglutide (3 mg) after 1 year of treatment resulted in mean decrease of 8% body weight. Approximately two-thirds of patients treated with liraglutide achieved >5% and one third achieved >10% weight loss.[3] Daily dosing of semaglutide at 2.4 mg achieved >15% weight loss in 50% of the study participants, whereas >20% weight loss was experienced by one-third of the study population.[3] Decrease in weight with semaglutide is more obvious in PCOS women with type 2 diabetes. With the use of orlistat, the mean total body weight loss was 10.6 kg at the end of one year. The compliance with orlistat was about 93% with an overall dropout rate of 8%.[3]

Phentermine/topiramate is used in the dose of 3.75 mg/23 mg or 15 mg/92 mg. In a study conducted where phentermine/topiramate was used with a reduced calorie diet for 56 weeks the weight reduction seen was 8.6% for the low-dose group and 8.5% for the high-dose group.[4] Recently released Indian Society for Assisted Reproduction (ISAR) guidelines mandate the offering of antiobesity drugs to women who present with infertility with BMI of ≥27 without comorbidities or ≥30 with comorbidities.[5]

Combinations of antiobesity medication may be necessary if one reaches a plateau of weight loss with one type of drug. For example, a patient who has lost weight with metformin and reached a weight loss plateau may experience increased hunger due to higher levels of ghrelin; then in these cases, one could use an appetite suppressant such as phentermine or phentermine/topiramate.[6]

Research gap: Large randomized controlled trials in women from different parts of the world and India comparing the efficacy of currently available medications are as yet awaited. Some combinations have been tried in clinical trials but others have not been tested in RCTs and have been used at the clinicians' discretion.[6]

5.3.2. Are antiobesity medications effective as per the evidence from large clinical trials, systematic reviews and meta-analyses?

Draft recommendations:

5.3.2.1. The currently available antiobesity medications are effective in the management of obesity in women and result in at least 5% weight loss at the end of 1 year of treatment. *(Moderate quality of evidence)*

Evidence: A systematic review and meta-analysis by Wang F et al. published 2018 included 941 women from 23 trials who had obesity (BMI >28 kg/m^2) and PCOS. The amount of weight lost differed significantly among the drugs (in descending order): Liraglutide, orlistat and metformin. Liraglutide alone, liraglutide/metformin and metformin alone significantly reduced waist circumference (–5.69, –4.68 and –2.68), but no change was found with orlistat.[7]

Rubino D et al. conducted the double blind, randomized 68-week STEP-4 trial at 73 sites in 10 countries from June 2018 to March 2020 in adults with body mass index of at least 30 (or ≥27 with ≥1 weight-related comorbidity) and without diabetes. 902 participants received once-weekly subcutaneous semaglutide during run-in. After 20 weeks, 89% participants who reached the 2.4 mg/week semaglutide maintenance dose were randomized (2:1) to 48 weeks of continued subcutaneous semaglutide (n = 535) or switched to placebo (n = 268), plus lifestyle intervention in both groups. Among the participants who completed a 20-week run-in period with subcutaneous semaglutide 2.4 mg once weekly, maintaining treatment with semaglutide compared with switching to placebo resulted in continued weight loss over the following 48 weeks.[8]

A systematic literature review and meta-analysis of 28 randomized controlled trials including over 29,000 participants published in JAMA in 2016 found that all of the above drugs/combinations are associated with significantly greater weight loss after 1 year when compared to placebo. The researchers concluded that the weight loss for each was approximately 5.3 kg (liraglutide) and 2.6 kg (orlistat). Discontinuation rates were highest with liraglutide and orlistat had the least side effects.[9]

Another meta-analysis published in 2020 found a significant reduction in body weight with orlistat (–3.07 kg) and liraglutide (–5.25 kg) when compared to placebo ($p < 0.00001$).[10]

In April 2021, the EMA has authorized the use of liraglutide for the treatment of obesity in adolescents (12–17 years). In the largest randomized clinical trial conducted on adolescents with obesity where liraglutide 3 mg was administered, all the participants also received lifestyle therapy and the mean BMI reduction was approximately 5% at the end of one year of treatment. More participants in the liraglutide group had a decline in BMI by 5% (43.3% liraglutide vs. 18.7% placebo) and 10% (26.1% liraglutide vs. 8.1% placebo).[11]

Research gaps: Randomized clinical trials of the new generation of antiobesity drugs in Indian obese PCOS women is currently lacking.

5.3.3. What are the advantages and disadvantages of the antiobesity agents currently available?

Draft recommendations:

5.3.3.1. Use of orlistat is associated with oily rectal leakage, abdominal distress, abdominal pain, flatulence with discharge, fecal urgency, steatorrhea, fecal incontinence, and increased defecation. *(Very low quality of evidence)*

5.3.3.2. The use of liraglutide is associated with increased heart rate, hypoglycemia, constipation, diarrhea, nausea, vomiting, and headache. *(Low quality of evidence)*

5.3.3.3. The use of semaglutide is associated with nausea, vomiting, diarrhea, abdominal pain, constipation, and headache. *(Very low quality of evidence)*

5.3.3.4. Use of phentermine/topiramate is associated with elevation in heart rate, mood and sleep disorders, cognitive impairment, metabolic acidosis, paresthesia, and dry mouth. *(Very low quality of evidence)*

Summary of evidence: Orlistat works by inhibiting the enzyme lipase in the mucous membranes of the stomach, small intestine and pancreas which results in preventing the conversion of triglycerides from ingested food into fatty acids and blocking absorption of about 30% of triglycerides in the intestine. Orlistat is efficacious in inducing at least 5% weight loss in 21% of patients, while 12% achieve 10% or greater weight loss when taken for a year. The side effects of orlistat which are experienced by about 20% patients are directly related to its principal action and include fecal incontinence, oily spotting, and fatty stools. Some patients with obesity who take orlistat and suddenly go on a concurrent diet may experience severe constipation owing to reduced amounts of dietary fiber in their food. Hence, dietary fiber supplementation is recommended for these patients along with orlistat. Malabsorption syndrome with lowered absorption of the fat soluble vitamins A, D, E, and K can occur, which needs exogenous supplementation. Owing to increased concentrations of oxalic acid in the urine, renal calculi may occasionally occur, though these are rare occurrences.[12]

Orlistat is widely recognized as one of the safest antiobesity drugs even in adolescents as only a small amount of drug is absorbed into the circulation. Large clinical trials have shown significant weight loss from the baseline when compared to placebo after 1 year and such weight loss has been maintained after 4 years of being on orlistat.

A risk reduction of 37% in the incidence of diabetes has been documented (XENDOS study). A meta-analysis published in the BMJ which included 30 randomized clinical trials reported that 21% of patients on orlistat for at least 1 year achieve at least 5% weight loss while 12% achieved weight loss of 10% or greater when compared to placebo.[12,13]

The newest class of antiobesity drugs is glucagon-like peptide-1 (GLP-1) agonists of which liraglutide and semaglutide are the prominent members. GLP-1 is secreted in humans after a carbohydrate and fat meal and triggers satiety, reducing further caloric intake. Liraglutide is 97% similar in structure to naturally occurring human GLP-1, with the critical difference that its action lasts longer than the natural variant.

It acts on the GLP-1 receptors situated in the hypothalamus leading to stimulation of transcript neurons which are sensitive to POMC, cocaine and amphetamines. The end result is appetite suppression. It also indirectly inhibits other neurons including neuropeptide-Y neurons which usually stimulate appetite. It also delays gastric emptying and regulates the balance between insulin and glucagon. Thus, it is responsible for weight loss via appetite suppression and its peripheral actions.[14]

The primary side effects of liraglutide include gastrointestinal symptoms including diarrhea, nausea, constipation and vomiting; the dose should be gradually increased to reduce the incidence of such side effects. Liraglutide therapy is associated with tachycardia, gallstones and pancreatitis. There are concerns about its association with medullary thyroid cancer and multiple endocrine neoplasia; hence, it is contraindicated in patients with a past or family history of such conditions. Multiple studies over the past few years have firmly established GLP-1 agonists as some of the best available agents for sustained weight loss, especially in subjects with comorbidities. A series of four trials labeled SCALE—Satiety and Clinical Adiposity Liraglutide investigated the safety and efficacy of liraglutide 3.0 mg compared with placebo in combination with a low-calorie diet and increased physical activity.

The mean weight loss was significantly higher in the liraglutide group when compared to placebo (8.4 vs. 2.8 kg, 6.4 vs. 2.2 kg, 6.2% vs. 0.2%). Significantly more patients on liraglutide achieved at least 5% weight loss (63% vs. 27%, 54% vs. 21%, 50% vs. 22%). In the entire series of trials, liraglutide demonstrated immense benefit as regards glycemic control, lowering of blood pressure, improving lipid levels and health-related quality of life in overweight or obese subjects.[15-17]

In patients with obesity with moderate or severe obstructive sleep apnea (OSA) given liraglutide 3.0 mg, after 32 weeks the apnea-hypopnea index (AHI) was significantly lower when compared to placebo (–12 events/h vs. –6.1 events/h). It has also been shown to improve hepatic steatosis in patients with non-alcoholic steatohepatitis. In women with PCOS, liraglutide therapy has resulted in 5.2 kg weight loss over 26 weeks of treatment.[18,19]

Research gaps: Currently, orlistat and liraglutide and oral preparation of semaglutide are available in India. Head-to-head comparisons between the three drugs are still awaited. One of the main challenges in weight management is the inability to predict patient's response to medications, as they respond differently to the antiobesity medications.

5.3.4. What are the contraindications for using antiobesity medicine?

Draft recommendations:

5.3.4.1. Antiobesity drugs can be used as long as there is no contraindication for their use and do not result in significant side-effects. *(Low quality of evidence)*

Summary of evidence: In general, contraindications for the use of antiobesity medications are post-bariatric surgery weight regain, depression, anxiety, severe mental illness, eating disorders, individuals of child-bearing potential, and elderly patients.[6]

TABLE 1: Contraindications of antiobesity medications.

Antiobesity medication	*Contraindications*
Orlistat	Chronic malabsorption syndrome or cholestasis, pregnancy
Phentermine/ topiramate	Glaucoma, hyperthyroidism, during or within 14 days following the administration of monoamine oxidase inhibitors, hypersensitivity to sympathomimetic amines, pregnancy
Liraglutide	Personal or family history of medullary thyroid carcinoma or multiple endocrine neoplasia syndrome type 2, pregnancy
Semaglutide	Personal or family history of medullary thyroid carcinoma or multiple endocrine neoplasia syndrome type 2, pregnancy

The specific contraindications for the use of antiobesity medications are given in the **Table 1**.[2]

Research gap: Today, obesity has become one of the chronic diseases. Further research is necessary on the assessment of cost-effectiveness, and tolerability, to determine effective treatment options, along with the study of the relationship with the existing contraindications for the use of antiobesity medications for long-term use.

5.3.5. How long should the antiobesity drugs be administered?

Draft recommendation:

5.3.5.1. The length of time one takes antiobesity drugs depends on weight loss and whether one experiences any serious side effects. *(Clinical practice point)*

Summary of evidence: If the patients are able to lose at least 5% of body weight with experiencing serious side-effects after taking the full dose of a drug for 3–6 months, its long-term use is justified.

If a 5% weight loss is not seen after the use of antiobesity medication for 3 months, one has to either stop the medication or change the treatment plan.[6] The last option is to refer to a bariatric surgeon for bariatric surgery. One must also remember that there is some amount of weight gain after stopping taking weight management medication. Life style modification with a healthy diet and regular physical activity will help in preventing weight gain and if it occurs it is minimal.[6]

Research gap: Most studies are retrospective and done without controls who are managed with lifestyle interventions alone.

CONCLUSION

Management of obesity should aim at achieving clinically significant weight loss and preventing the development or exacerbation of comorbid conditions. If lifestyle modification is unable to achieve desired weight loss and the comorbidities are significantly high antiobesity medication is necessary to achieve effective weight loss. As direct comparative clinical studies are lacking for the antiobesity medication, their use is based on relative efficacy and safety.

REFERENCES

1. Swinburn BA, Kraak VI, Allender S, et al. The global syndemic of obesity, undernutrition, and climate change: the Lancet Commission report. Lancet. 2019;393:791-846.
2. Chakhtoura M, Haber R, Ghezzawi M, et al. Pharmacotherapy of obesity: an update on the available medications and drugs under investigation. EClinicalMedicine. 2023;58:101882.
3. Müller TD, Blüher M, Tschöp MH, et al. Anti-obesity drug discovery: advances and challenges. Nat Rev Drug Discov. 2022;21(3):201-23.
4. Allison DB, Gadde KM, Garvey WT, et al. Controlled-release phentermine/topiramate in severely obese adults: a randomized controlled trial (EQUIP). Obesity (Silver Spring). 2012;20(2):330-42.
5. Palshetkar N, Pai H, Patel M, et al. Optimizing obesity management for women in an Indian obstetrics and gynecology setting: a consensus approach by the Indian Society of Assisted Reproduction (ISAR). Indian J Obstet Gynecol Res. 2024;11(3):330-44.
6. Weintraub MA, D'Angelo D, Tchang BG, et al. Five-year weight loss maintenance with obesity pharmacotherapy. J Clin Endocrinol Metab. 2023;108(9):e832-41.
7. Wang FF, Wu Y, Zhu YH, et al. Pharmacologic therapy to induce weight loss in women who have obesity/overweight with polycystic ovary syndrome: a systematic review and network meta-analysis. Obes Rev. 2018;19(10):1424-45.
8. Rubino D, Abrahamsson N, Davies M, et al.; STEP 4 Investigators. Effect of continued weekly subcutaneous semaglutide vs placebo on weight loss maintenance in adults with overweight or obesity: the STEP 4 randomized clinical trial. JAMA. 2021;325(14):1414-25.
9. Khera R, Pandey A, Chandar AK, et al. Effects of weight-loss medications on cardiometabolic risk profiles: a systematic review and network meta-analysis. Gastroenterology. 2018;154(5):1309-19.e7.
10. Singh AK, Singh R. Pharmacotherapy in obesity: a systematic review and meta-analysis of randomized controlled trials of anti-obesity drugs. Expert Rev Clin Pharmacol. 2020;13(1):53-64.
11. Kelly AS, Auerbach P, Barrientos-Perez M, et al. A randomized, controlled trial of liraglutide for adolescents with obesity. N Engl J Med. 2020;382:2117-28.
12. Rucker D, Padwal R, Li SK, et al. Long term pharmacotherapy for obesity and overweight: updated meta-analysis. BMJ. 2007;335:1194-9.
13. Torgerson JS, Hauptman J, Boldrin MN, et al. XENical in the prevention of diabetes in obese subjects (XENDOS) study: a randomized study of orlistat as

an adjunct to lifestyle changes for the prevention of type 2 diabetes in obese patients. Diabetes Care. 2004;27:155-61.
14. Barrera JG, Sandoval DA, D'Alessio DA, et al. GLP-1 and energy balance: an integrated model of short-term and long-term control. Nat Rev Endocrinol. 2011;7:507-16.
15. Pi-Sunyer X, Astrup A, Fujioka K, et al.; SCALE Obesity and Prediabetes NN8022-1839 Study Group. A randomized, controlled trial of 3.0 mg of liraglutide in weight management. N Engl J Med. 2015;373:11-22.
16. Davies MJ, Bergenstal R, Bode B, et al.; NN8022-1922 Study Group. Efficacy of liraglutide for weight loss among patients with type 2 diabetes: the SCALE diabetes randomized clinical trial. JAMA. 2015;314:687-99.
17. Wadden TA, Hollander P, Klein S, et al.; NN8022-1923 Investigators. Weight maintenance and additional weight loss with liraglutide after low-calorie-diet-induced weight loss: the SCALE maintenance randomized study. Int J Obes (Lond). 2013;37:1443-51.
18. Blackman A, Foster GD, Zammit G, et al. Effect of liraglutide 3.0 mg in individuals with obesity and moderate or severe obstructive sleep apnea: the SCALE sleep apnea randomized clinical trial. Int J Obes (Lond). 2016;40:1310-9.
19. Nylander M, Frossing S, Clausen HV, et al. Effects of liraglutide on ovarian dysfunction in polycystic ovary syndrome: a randomized clinical trial. Reprod Biomed Online. 2017;35:121-7.

5.4 ROLE OF BARIATRIC SURGERY IN PCOS

Rajsekhar Nayak, Rajesh Pendlimari, Nagesh NS

INTRODUCTION

At least one-third of the population is overweight or obese and 50% of the PCOS women are obese. Obesity adversely affects fertility and psychological health and increases the risk of metabolic disorders.[1-3] Weight loss improves outcomes for all symptoms associated with PCOS. The role of bariatric surgery is increasingly recognized in the management of obese PCOS patients. It provides substantial and lasting weight loss with improvement in health and well-being. Most guidelines recommend surgery to aid weight loss for women with BMI >35 kg/m^2 or for a BMI between 30 and 34.9 kg/m^2 with associated metabolic comorbidity.

A large percentage of patients undergoing bariatric surgery belong to the reproductive age group. Follow-up of these patients has thrown light on the physiological changes that take place including that on the reproductive system after bariatric surgery.

The commonly performed procedures are laparoscopic sleeve gastrectomy (LSG) and Roux-en-Y gastric bypass (RYGB). The newer modification of RYGB which is called mini gastric bypass or one anastomosis gastric bypass has been gaining prominence in recent years. There are no comparative studies between the various procedures in lieu of the advantage for PCOS. The choice of bariatric surgery procedure for PCOS patients should be based on surgeon preference and patients' comorbidities.

5.4.1. Is bariatric/metabolic surgery effective for the management of hormonal and clinical PCOS features and weight?

Draft recommendations:

5.4.1.1. Bariatric surgery in the forms of LSG and RYGB is effective in normalizing metabolic parameters such as triglycerides, fasting glucose, fasting insulin, HOMA-IR, HbA1C but also improving SHBG, lowering testosterone and free androgen index. *(Low quality of evidence)*

5.4.1.2. The effect on AMH levels is conflicting. *(Very low quality of evidence)*

Summary of evidence: Bariatric surgery significantly improved hormonal and metabolic parameters in obese PCOS patients. A meta-analysis of 21 studies demonstrated significant decrease in testosterone levels, fasting glucose, insulin and triglycerides after bariatric surgery. There is greater weight loss and reduction in HOMA-IR after surgery as compared to conservative treatment in women with and without PCOS. Menstrual cycles became regular and ovulatory in those women who underwent surgery.[4]

In a prospective non-RCT study of 81 women with PCOS, LSG was compared with metformin therapy. There was significant weight loss and decrease in waist-hip ratio, androgen levels, fasting insulin, HOMA-IR, HbA1C levels, triglycerides, LDL-cholesterol and an increase in SHBG and insulin sensitivity in the surgical group.[5] Decreased inflammation, hyperandrogenemia and hyperinsulinemia and an increase in adiponectin post bariatric surgery improve ovulation rates and restore menstrual function.[6]

Data regarding AMH levels after weight loss strategies is conflicting. Some studies have shown a significantly increased AMH in 6 months after surgery while others have shown a significant decrease in AMH levels[7,8] at 12 months.[6] Bariatric surgery was associated with improvement in quality of life and reduction in mental disorders.[6] Female sexual dysfunction, measured with female sexual functional index (FSFI) questionnaire showed that desire and arousal significantly increased after bariatric surgery.

The BAMBINI trial is the only RCT[9] that evaluated the safety and efficacy of bariatric surgery in comparison to medical therapy in women with PCOS, obesity and oligomenorrhea or amenorrhea. A total of 80 women were recruited and randomized to either laparoscopic sleeve gastrectomy or medical management including behavioral interventions and medical therapy. The incidence of spontaneous ovulation was 2.5 times more in the surgical group compared to medical therapy ($p < 0.0007$). There was a significant decrease in weight, waist circumference, free androgen index,

HbA1C, blood pressure, fasting glucose, fasting insulin, triglycerides and HOMA-IR. There was a significant difference in the free androgen index even at 52 weeks. There was a significant reduction in the AMH levels in the surgical group, but the difference was not significant at 52 weeks. There was a significant improvement in PCOSQ score and HADS depression score in the surgical group. There was a higher incidence of folic acid deficiency in the surgical group. BAMBINI RCT showed that LSG was superior to medical management.[9]

Research gaps: There were not many randomized controlled trials that assessed the impact of bariatric surgery on PCOS. There are no studies that have done direct comparison between medical therapy (clomiphene, inositols or GLP-1 analogs such as semaglutide) and bariatric surgery. Also, there are no studies that have compared the efficacy of different surgical techniques for bariatric surgery.

5.4.2. What are the indications for bariatric Surgery in adolescents and adults?

Draft recommendations:

5.4.2.1. For adolescents, bariatric surgery should be considered after evaluation by a multidisciplinary team in the presence of overweight (BMI is at or above the 85th percentile and below the 97th percentile) or severe obesity (BMI above the 97th percentile) and those who have previously participated in lifestyle interventions with unsuccessful outcomes. *(Low quality of evidence)*

- Class II obesity—BMI >120% of the 95th percentile with comorbidity
- Class III obesity—BMI >140% of the 95th percentile

5.4.2.2. In adults bariatric surgery should be considered depending on the BMI and presence or absence of comorbidities. *(Low quality of evidence)*

- Obese—BMI >35 kg/m^2 regardless of comorbidities
- BMI >30 kg/m^2 with type 2 diabetes mellitus
- Class I obesity—BMI of 30–34.9 kg/m^2 who do not achieve substantial or durable weight loss or comorbidity improvement using nonsurgical methods

5.4.2.3. Bariatric surgery is not recommended for PCOS per se. *(Clinical practice point)*

Summary of evidence: ASMBS pediatric metabolic and bariatric surgery guidelines, 2018[10] use the following definitions for childhood obesity: (1) BMI cut-offs of 35 kg/m^2 or 120% of the 95th percentile with a comorbidity, or (2) BMI >40 kg/m^2 or 140% of the 95th percentile without a comorbidity (whichever is less). Earlier surgical intervention when BMI is <45 kg/m^2 can avoid lifelong medication therapy and prevent end organ damage from comorbidities in adolescents. Moreover, certain comorbidities like the psychosocial burden of obesity, orthopedic diseases specific to children, GERD, and cardiac risk factors should be considered as an indication for bariatric surgery in adolescents. As medical therapies have a poor outcome in children and adolescents with T2D, it should be considered an indication for bariatric surgery despite lower obesity percentiles. The decision for bariatric surgery in adolescents should be taken only after evaluation by a multidisciplinary team in a speciality center.[2]

Bariatric surgery is recommended for individuals with a body mass index (BMI) > 35 kg/m^2, regardless of presence, absence, or severity of comorbidities. It should also be considered for individuals with a BMI of 30–34.9 kg/m^2 with metabolic disease. It is important that we must adjust BMI thresholds in the Asian population as BMI of 25 kg/m^2 suggests clinical obesity, and therefore individuals with BMI of 27.5 kg/m^2 should be offered bariatric surgery.[2]

PCOS per se is not an indication for any bariatric surgery though it improves the metabolic and reproductive outcomes of PCOS in women with obesity. The efficacy and safety of surgery on PCOS have to be evaluated in a randomized trial. As obesity exacerbates subfertility in PCOS women, bariatric surgery in overweight and obese PCOS improves weight loss, hirsutism, irregular menstrual cycles, ovulation, and pregnancy rates.[6] Bhandari et al. conducted a prospective study in more than 1000 PCOS women with 5-year follow-up and observed that LAGB led to 32% weight loss at 5 years, 93% women had regular menstrual cycles at 6 months and a significant reduction in hirsutism.[11] Another prospective study found significant weight loss, resumption of regular menstrual cycle and decreased hirsutism in both PCOS and non-PCOS women following bariatric procedure.[12] Seven out of 14 women had complete resolution of ovarian polycystic morphology on ultrasound at the end of 1 year.[12]

BAMBINI trial is the only randomized control trial to prove the superiority of bariatric surgery (LSG) over medical management in improving the fertility.[9] Regardless of fertility markers, bariatric surgery increased pregnancy rate in nulliparous women.

There are no studies that assessed the impact of bariatric surgery for PCOS women on outcomes of ART (assisted reproductive technology). In a retrospective study, post-bariatric surgery, 25% of infertile women conceived with ART.[13] This indicated that bariatric surgery may improve the success of ART. RYGB is the most effective procedure as it significantly reduces weight and corrects metabolic syndrome.

Research gaps: Recommendations for bariatric surgery in adolescent and adult PCOS have limited evidence. The current guidelines do not recommend bariatric surgery for all women with PCOS, but may have a beneficial effect in an obese PCOS. The most effective procedure has not yet been evaluated in terms of infertility secondary to PCOS.

5.4.3. What are the maternal and fetal complications of bariatric surgery?

Draft recommendations:

5.4.3.1. Bariatric surgery may result in nutritional deficiencies, anemia, altered maternal glucose metabolism and small for gestational age children, which may then result in adverse outcomes both in the mother and neonate. Women are therefore counseled to use effective contraception immediately before surgery or after surgery to delay conception for 1–1.5 years to prevent maternal and neonatal complications. *(Low quality of evidence)*

5.4.3.2. Bariatric surgeries may significantly reduce the occurrence of obesity-related complications during pregnancy like GDM, PIH, PE, and CSs. *(Moderate quality of evidence)*

5.4.3.3. Maternal and perinatal outcomes differ according to type of bariatric surgery and serious surgical complications are more common with gastric bypass than gastric banding. Therefore the choice of bariatric surgery should take into account the impact of surgery on future pregnancy. *(Low quality of evidence)*

Summary of evidence: Obese-pregnant women are at increased risk of developing GDM, pregnancy-induced hypertension (PIH), preeclampsia (PE), and cesarean sections (CSs).[14] Bariatric surgeries may significantly reduce the occurrence of obesity-related complications during pregnancy like GDM, PIH, PE, and CSs. Protein, iron, folate, calcium, and vitamin B12 and D are the most common nutritional deficiencies seen after gastric bypass surgery, which may have a negative effect on the fetus. These deficiencies can increase the risk of neural tube defects but not other congenital anomalies. If pregnancy occurs in less than 18 months after BS or if the neonate was small for gestational age at birth, the prevalence of neurodevelopmental disorders was significantly higher.[15] Bariatric surgery may result in small for gestational age (SGA) fetuses and intrauterine growth restriction (IUGR) of infants due to maternal malnutrition and micronutrient deficiency.[12,14] Higher incidence of perinatal mortality and preterm birth was also reported.[16] Therefore regular follow-up with blood examinations and ultrasound for growth curve, umbilical Doppler and amniotic fluid index) are necessary.[14]

The oral glucose-tolerance testing could be unsafe owing to the risk of the dumping syndrome (i.e., rapid gastric emptying) after bariatric surgery. These women therefore are advised to assess fasting glucose levels and preprandial and postprandial glucose values instead.[17]

Women pregnant after gastric banding and sleeve gastrectomy had a lower risk of anemia and gestational diabetes compared with gastric bypass.[18] Infants had a higher birth weight if they were born after gastric banding rather than gastric bypass or sleeve gastrectomy. The risk of preterm birth was higher in women with gastric banding as compared with gastric bypass.[18] One study concluded that maternal (17.6 vs. 22.2%, $p = 0.843$) and neonatal (23.5 vs. 14.8%, $p = 0.466$) complications were reported to be rare, and no significant difference was observed between PCOS women and non-PCOS women.[19] Ideally all pregnant patients who have undergone bariatric surgery should be referred to a multidisciplinary team with experience in the management of pregnancies after BS.

Research gaps: Though we clearly understand the consequences of bariatric surgery such as vitamin and mineral deficiencies good data is lacking about the outcomes of bariatric surgery in terms of maternal and fetal complications. There is no international treatment consensus for pregnancy after BS, hence specific recommendations are not yet available. This creates an extreme challenge for the treating obstetrician.

The data of women undergoing bariatric surgery regardless of PCOS is available and the same data is extrapolated to obese women with PCOS.

5.4.4. Can bariatric surgery influence the fertility and pregnancy outcome?

Draft recommendations:

5.4.4.1. Bariatric surgery has a positive impact on the pregnancy with increased chance of spontaneous conception or a better success rate after ART. *(Low quality of evidence)*

5.4.4.2. Female sexual dysfunction (FSD) is resolved after bariatric surgery as assessed by female sexual function index (FSFI). *(Low quality of evidence)*

5.4.4.3. Little is known about the effect of bariatric surgery on breastfeeding, so it should not be restricted after bariatric surgery. *(Very low quality of evidence)*

Summary of evidence: A retrospective study by Nayak et al. compared PCOS and non-PCOS Indian women who underwent bariatric surgery. A total of 10 PCOS women out of 17 became pregnant, of which 9 women conceived spontaneously.[20] The average birth weight in the PCOS group was 2.58 kg, which was slightly higher than the non-PCOS group.[20]

A prospective study by Benito et al. compared PCOS women with non-PCOS women who underwent bariatric surgery (LAGB, LSG, or RYGB) and assessed pregnancy and outcomes.[19] 17 women with PCOS had at least one pregnancy, compared to controls ($\chi^2 = 4.643$, $p = 0.031$). Pregnancy rates were significantly higher (40.8% vs. 25%) in women with PCOS.[19] The number of newborns with low birth weight were similar in both groups.[19]

Another retrospective study from Christinajoice et al. compared PCOS and non-PCOS women after bariatric surgery.[21] Out of 45 patients studied, 19 patients conceived and had a live birth. Pre-term births occurred in 63% and full-term births in 37% of the women. Small for gestational age babies (≤2.5 kg) were born to 19 women (47.3%) with mean body weight of 2.13 ± 0.8 kg. Fourteen (73.6%) patients had a normal delivery, whereas 5 (26.3%) patients underwent a cesarean section.[21] The incidence of maternal anemia was 36.8%. There was no increased incidence of gestational diabetes and PIH or congenital anomalies in the offspring.

Bariatric surgery resolves the sexual dysfunction in women less than 40 years old for at least 1 year post-surgery. The beneficial effect of bariatric surgery on sexual function beyond 1 year still needs to be verified.[22]

Though some studies in the past have reported failure to thrive in the newborn, recent studies have shown that the composition of breast milk after bariatric surgery was found to be comparable with women without bariatric surgery. Despite that it is recommended to continue nutritional supplements during the period of breastfeeding.[23]

Research gaps: Few small cohort studies have shown a positive impact of bariatric surgery on the occurrence of pregnancy spontaneously or after ART. But currently, there is a lack of trials that compare the efficacy of bariatric surgery in reducing pregnancy complications and improving the success of ART in comparison with obesity pharmacotherapy. This information needs to be confirmed with a randomized control trial.

CONCLUSION

Obesity exacerbates the manifestations of PCOS. Weight loss forms the crux of management in these patients. Lifestyle modifications along with medical management (metformin and inositols) are the first-line therapies in the management of these patients targeting weight loss. Though GLP-1 analogues are increasingly showing promise, a clear-cut evidence is still awaited. BS appears to be an effective long-term weight-loss solution with improved ovulation and fertility and reduced pregnancy comorbidities. It also addresses metabolic and hormonal dysfunction. The surgical technique used, and the long-term safety and effect on neonates and children are yet to be established as surgery can cause nutrient deficiencies important for fetal development. Further RCTs are required to establish the efficacy and safety of bariatric surgery in women with PCOS.

REFERENCES

1. Wang R, Kim BV, van Wely M, et al. Treatment strategies for women with WHO group II anovulation: systematic review and network meta-analysis. BMJ. 2017;356:j138.

2. Eisenberg D, Shikora SA, Aarts E, et al. 2022 American Society for Metabolic and Bariatric Surgery (ASMBS) and International Federation for the Surgery of obesity and metabolic disorders (IFSO): indications for metabolic and bariatric surgery. Surg Obes Relat Dis. 2022;18(12):1345-56.
3. Tian Z, Zhang YC, Wang Y, et al. Effects of bariatric surgery on patients with obesity and polycystic ovary syndrome: a meta-analysis. Surg Obes Relat Dis. 2021;17(8):1399-408.
4. Tatarchuk T, Todurov I, Anagnostis P, et al. The effect of gastric sleeve resection on menstrual pattern and ovulation in premenopausal women with classes III–IV obesity. Obes Surg. 2022;32(3):599-606.
5. Hu L, Ma L, Xia X, et al. Efficacy of bariatric surgery in the treatment of women with obesity and polycystic ovary syndrome. J Clin Endocrinol Metab. 2022;107(8):e3217-29.
6. Samarasinghe SNS, Woods C, Miras AD. Bariatric surgery in women with polycystic ovary syndrome. Metabolism. 2023;151:155745.
7. Chiofalo F, Ciuoli C, Formichi C, et al. Bariatric surgery reduces serum anti-mullerian hormone levels in obese women with and without polycystic ovarian syndrome. Obes Surg. 2017;27(7):1750-4.
8. Nilsson-Condori E, Hedenbro JL, Thurin-Kjellberg A, et al. Impact of diet and bariatric surgery on anti-Müllerian hormone levels. Hum Reprod. 2018;33(4):690-3.
9. Samarasinghe SNS, Leca B, Alabdulkader S, et al. Bariatric surgery for spontaneous ovulation in women living with polycystic ovary syndrome: the BAMBINI multicentre, open-label, randomised controlled trial. Lancet. 2024;403(10443):2489-503.
10. Pratt JS, Browne A, Browne NT, et al. ASMBS pediatric metabolic and bariatric surgery guidelines, 2018. Surg Obes Relat Dis. 2018;14(7):882-901.
11. Bhandari M, Kosta S, Bhandari M, et al. Effects of bariatric surgery on people with obesity and polycystic ovary syndrome: a large single center study from India. Obes Surg. 2022;32(10):3305-12.
12. Singh D, Arumalla K, Aggarwal S, et al. Impact of bariatric surgery on clinical, biochemical, and hormonal parameters in women with polycystic ovary syndrome (PCOS). Obes Surg. 2020;30(6):2294-300.
13. Nilsson-Condori E, Mattsson K, Thurin-Kjellberg A, et al. Outcomes of in-vitro fertilization after bariatric surgery: a national register-based case–control study. Hum Reprod. 2022;37(10):2474-81.
14. Falcone V, Stopp T, Feichtinger M, et al. Pregnancy after bariatric surgery: a narrative literature review and discussion of impact on pregnancy management and outcome. BMC Pregnancy Childbirth. 2018;18:507.
15. Micic DD, Toplak H, Micic DD, et al. Reproductive outcomes after bariatric surgery in women. Wien Klin Wochenschrift. 2022;134(1):56-62.
16. Akhter Z, Rankin J, Ceulemans D, et al. Pregnancy after bariatric surgery and adverse perinatal outcomes: a systematic review and meta-analysis. PLoS Med. 2019;16(8):e1002866.
17. Johansson K, Cnattingius S, Näslund I, et al. Outcomes of pregnancy after bariatric surgery. N Engl J Med. 2015;372(9):814-24.
18. Cornthwaite K, Prajapati C, Lenguerrand E, et al. Pregnancy outcomes following different types of bariatric surgery: a national cohort study. Eur J Obstet Gynecol Reprod Biol. 2021;260:10-7.

19. Benito E, GÓmez-Martin JM, Vega-Piñero B, et al. Fertility and pregnancy outcomes in women with polycystic ovary syndrome following bariatric surgery. J Clin Endocrinol Metab. 2020;105 (9):e3384-91.
20. Nayak R, Gunasheela D, Kumar V, et al. Effectiveness of bariatric surgery-induced weight loss on infertility among PCOS and non-PCOS women: experience of a maternity hospital and in vitro fertilization (IVF) center in India. Indian J Surg. 2020;6:1-7.
21. Christinajoice S, Misra S, Bhattacharya S, et al. Impact of bariatric surgery on female reproductive health and maternal outcomes. Obes Surg. 2020;30(2):383-90.
22. Loh HH, Shahar MA, Loh HS, et al. Female sexual dysfunction after bariatric surgery in women with obesity: a systematic review and meta-analysis. Scand J Surg. 2022;111(1):14574969211072395.
23. Mokhlesi SS, Vasilevski V, Sweet L. Breastfeeding and pre-pregnancy bariatric surgery: a scoping review. Women Birth. 2024;37(3):101600.

5.5 COMMON SLEEP DISORDERS IN POLYCYSTIC OVARY SYNDROME

Suma P Kumar, Darsana G, Danne Shaji Philip

INTRODUCTION

Sleep is an important reparative process in human life. We spend approximately a third of our lives asleep. Anything that adversely affects it can have serious impact on our lives. Polycystic ovary syndrome (PCOS) with its associated features of obesity, hyperandrogenism, and hormonal imbalances can seriously affect sleep in these women in the prime of their lives. It is associated with adverse cardiometabolic effects, type 2 diabetes mellitus, nonalcoholic steatohepatitis and mood disorders. Associated sleep disorders are also common in these women and many a time, mood disorders may be implicated in their sleep complaints and an adequate assessment may not happen if one is not aware. Sleep disruption leads to increased visceral adiposity and insulin resistance which are also key factors noted in PCOS. The associated sleep disturbances can also contribute to the lifestyle behaviors observed in PCOS.[1] The common sleep disorders in PCOS include snoring and OSA (obstructive sleep apnea), insomnia, and restless legs. This review addresses these common sleep problems in PCOS, their pathophysiology, clinical and sleep evaluation methods along with treatment aspects.

METHODS

For each PICO question, using specific terms, MEDLINE and Cochrane database search was carried out. Although in the last decade there are many publications pertaining to PCOS, sleep disorders in PCOS has sparse literature with respect to prevalence, specific evaluation and treatment.

Relevant articles were read and GRADE system was used for analysis of PICO questions. Quality of grading was very low, low, moderate and high (e.g., data from randomized controlled trials will be graded as high evidence).

5.5.1. What are the PCOS effects on sleep?

Draft recommendations:

5.5.1.1. PCOS has an adverse effect on the sleep quality and thereby daytime functioning. *(Moderate to high quality of evidence)*

5.5.1.2. Sleep health evaluation to diagnose underlying sleep disorders especially OSA is essential. *(Moderate to high quality of evidence)*

Summary of evidence: In PCOS, there is a subjective perception of low quality of sleep and on sleep studies this has been demonstrated as reduced sleep efficiency (per cent time asleep), increased sleep latency (onset of sleep from time into bed), decreased time spent in rapid eye movement (REM) stage, increased number of obstructive respiratory events, and arousals that could all hamper daytime efficiency.[2] Long-term reduction in REM sleep translates to poor memory, inability to consolidate cognitive skills and increase in the risk of developing metabolic disorders. Increased obesity, visceral adiposity and changes in sex hormones (increased androgens and/or reduced estrogens) can all contribute to the associated sleep symptoms. However, studies have also shown that obstructive sleep apnea (OSA) in PCOS is independent of the level of obesity.

Research gaps:

1. There is a large gap in polysomnographic evidence of sleep disruption to subjective reports of poor quality of sleep and sleep disorders. Polysomnographic evaluation has to be evaluated in larger group of patients to objectively assess sleep parameters in PCOS.
2. Indian data has to be gathered to assess sleep quality both subjectively and objectively.

5.5.2. What is the pathophysiology of sleep disorders?

Draft recommendations:

5.5.2.1. Anatomic factors (such as micrognathia, large tongue as in acromegaly, hypothyroidism), large neck circumference, increased bony structures and soft tissues around the neck as seen in obesity increase the risk of obstructive sleep apnea (OSA). These features should be looked for in individual patients. *(Moderate to high quality of evidence)*

5.5.2.2. Upper airway collapsibility and pharyngeal narrowing is worsened by upper airway dilator hypo responsiveness, high loop gain, low arousal threshold and reduced ventilatory drive during sleep. *(Low to moderate quality of evidence)*

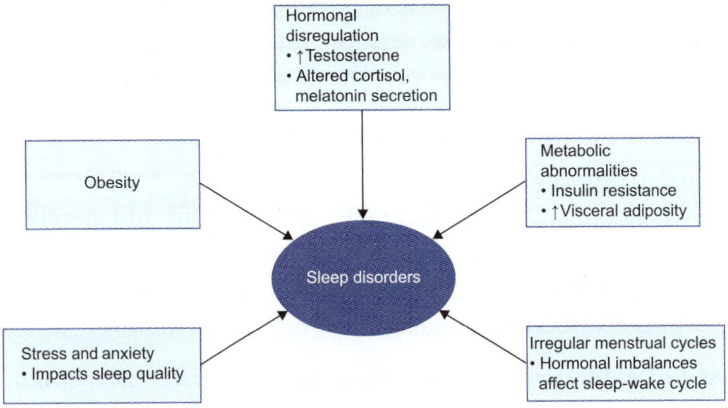

Fig. 1: Pathophysiology of various sleep disorders in PCOS.

Summary of evidence for etiopathogenesis of sleep disorders in PCOS (Fig. 1): The etiopathogenesis is multifactorial and a close relationship exists with the metabolic factors, OSA, and hormonal changes although the causal link is uncertain.

Research gaps: There is a close relationship between the mechanisms of OSA and PCOS in general. The specific mechanisms that contribute to each sleep disorder needs defined in PCOS.

5.5.3. What is the prevalence, evaluation and treatment options for snoring and OSA in PCOS?

Draft recommendations:

5.5.3.1. OSA forms the most common sleep disorder described in patients with PCOS. *(High quality of evidence)*

5.5.3.2. When there is a high clinical probability for OSA as assessed by symptoms and clinical evaluation including questionnaires, diagnosis should always be confirmed by sleep studies. *(High quality of evidence)*

5.5.3.3. Treatment options include lifestyle changes, continuous positive airway pressure therapy when severe or symptomatic and if that fails, consideration of a mandibular advancement device as in non-PCOS. *(Moderate quality of evidence)*

Summary of evidence:

Snoring and obstructive sleep apnea: Snoring prevalence is higher in PCOS. Most people snore occasionally and 25% are habitual snorers. Snoring was originally thought to be benign. However, there is evidence that there is increased association with vascular disease and reduced quality of life for snorers and their bed partners. Increased prevalence is noted in PCOS and they should be advised on lifestyle modifications, position therapy and if indicated, be evaluated for OSA as it can be a component of it.

OSA in women is much less common in premenopausal compared to postmenopausal women and men in general. However, in comparison to non PCOS group, PCOS patients are at a higher risk of snoring and sleep apnea.[1] Also, women are less likely to report the classical symptoms of OSA such as loud snoring, choking at night and daytime sleepiness. They are more likely to report tiredness, fatigue, insomnia, early morning headache, irritability—all of which can be attributed to PCOS or mood disorders. Although obesity is a risk factor for OSA, nonobese PCOS also have higher obstructive respiratory events, which suggest that the link between OSA and PCOS is not always due to obesity alone and the hormonal changes do contribute to the development of OSA in PCOS. Studies have shown that associated desaturations, high sympathetic tone and oxidative stress during apneas and hypopneas contributes to insulin resistance, which is also a hallmark of PCOS. The complex hormonal and metabolic changes of PCOS are closely intertwined with OSA. In a population-based UK cohort study with a median follow-up of 3.5 years (n = >200,000), OSA in PCOS showed higher incidence with an adjusted hazard ratio (HR) of 2.26, independent of BMI.[3]

Clinical evaluation: A comprehensive clinical assessment is mandatory prior to deciding on the type of sleep study that a patient needs for evaluation of their sleep symptoms. There may be the coexistence of other sleep disorders (e.g., restless legs). Neck circumference, body mass index (BMI), waist-to-hip ratio (>0.85 signifies abdominal obesity as per the World Health Organization) and airway narrowing (as per modified Mallampati score) will need to be assessed.

Body mass index is calculated from the ratio of weight to height squared **(Table 1)**. Considering metabolic diseases are higher in Asians compared to Caucasians, the Asian-Pacific recommendations for BMI targets a lower threshold for obesity in Asian origin people.

Sleepiness, clinical probability of sleep disorders and quality of sleep evaluation is carried out by questionnaires. The commonly used ones include Epworth sleepiness scale (8 questions assessing sleepiness on a scale to 0–3, a

TABLE 1: BMI classification.

BMI	*Classification*
18.5–22.9 kg/m^2	Normal
23–24.9 kg/m^2	Overweight
25–29.9 kg/m^2	Class I obesity
>30 kg/m^2	Class II obesity

score of ≥11 is considered excessive sleepiness), STOP BANG questionnaire, Pittsburg Sleep Quality Index (PSQI) and BERLIN questionnaires.

STOP-BANG questionnaire[4] is one of the widely used tool and a score of ≥3 signifies moderate-severe OSA risk. Each component gets a mark of 1 when answered yes. The components included are as follows:

- **S**noring: Loud **S**noring
- **T**iredness
- **O**bserved Apneas
- High Blood **P**ressure
- **B**MI > 35 kg/m^2
- **A**ge > 50 years
- **N**eck circumference> 40 cm (>17 inches in men and >16 inches in females)
- **G**ender: Male

Studies have shown that in PCOS patients, irrespective of obesity and hyperandrogenism, level of sleepiness as estimated by these questionnaires is high.

Sleep studies: Technician led, in-lab polysomnography (PSG, type I sleep study) remains the gold standard. **Table 2** summarizes the channels used in different levels of sleep studies as per the American Academy of Sleep Medicine (AASM). Types II-IV comprise the home sleep apnea testing (HSAT). There are only few studies that have evaluated sleep complaints in PCOS with PSG in the literature.[2]

When the patients present with classical symptoms with high clinical probability as assessed by physical examination and questionnaires, HSAT can be done in the comfort of patient's home. When multiple sleep disorders coexist or OSA clinical probability is low, type I study will be preferred.

Important sleep index:[6] Apnea hypopnea index (AHI)/respiratory event index (REI) in HSAT AHI is the total number of apneas and hypopneas recorded divided by the total sleep time. In REI, the denominator will be the total recording time (rather than the sleep time which is assessed by EEG in type I sleep study) and hence there is risk of underestimating the events. Severity of OSA is based on the AHI/REI.

AHI 5–14.9 events/hour: Mild OSA, 15–29.9/hour: Moderate OSA, ≥ 30: severe OSA.

Treatment: The underlying hormonal and metabolic imbalances should be addressed simultaneously. Treatment with continuous positive airway pressure (CPAP) therapy is initiated when patients are symptomatic and AHI ≥5 per hour or when AHI ≥15 even in absence of symptoms to improve quality of life and cardiometabolic issues.

Lifestyle modifications that are routinely helpful in PCOS such as weight reduction, physical activity and dietary modifications will also help in

TABLE 2: Types of sleep studies.[5]

	Type I (attended)	*Type II (unattended)*	*Type III (modified, for diagnosing OSA)*	*Type IV (1 or 2 channels)*
Measurement channels (n)	≥7	≥7	≥4	≤2
Measurements	Electroencephalogram Electrooculogram Chin electromyogram Electrocardiogram Air flow Respiratory effort Pulse oximetry	Electroencephalogram Electrooculogram Chin electromyogram Electrocardiogram Air flow Respiratory effort Pulse oximetry	Electrocardiogram Air flow Two respiratory-effort channels Pulse oximetry Peripheral arterial tonometry*	Pulse oximetry Air flow or chest movement
Body position	Documented or objective	Possible	Possible	No
Leg movement	Electromyogram or motion sensor	Optional	Optional	No
Personnel	Yes	No	No	No
Intervention	Possible	No	No	No

*Became available after 1994.

treatment of underlying sleep disorders especially OSA. Reassessment for the need of CPAP should be done when there is ≥10% body weight loss either attained through surgery or medical means.[7]

Oropharyngeal exercises, myofunctional therapy[8] and pranayama (such as Ujjayi breathing) have also shown to reduce sleepiness in mild-moderate OSA. Along with this, *sleep hygiene* plays an important role in all seeking good sleep and those experiencing sleep disturbances. The ten commandments of sleep hygiene include: regular exercise (not just before bedtime; morning or early evening is preferred), ensuring last meal of the day is at least 3 hours before sleep (if hungry just before bed, encourage to have milk or banana that is soporific), avoiding stimulants and caffeinated drinks (for at least 6 hours before bedtime), to ensure sleeping and wake up times are fixed (and at the same time; the circadian rhythm is most dependent on the wake up time), to use the bed only for sleep and sex, ensuring the bedroom has comfortable temperature (neither too hot or cold) and near-zero lighting, avoiding all screens for an hour before sleep (blue light emitted from the gadgets keeps us awake), watch your napping, avoiding alcohol and cigarettes.

Young patients with mild to moderate OSA who have failed CPAP therapy or unwilling to use the same can be advised to use *Mandibular advancement device (MAD)* at night to pull the jaw forward and create extra space to minimize the apneas. For maximal benefit, it must be custom made and titrated. Its benefit and place in treatment of PCOS associated OSA is yet to be determined.

Effects of drugs used in PCOS on sleep: Metformin used in PCOS has shown reduced sleepiness in adolescents;[9] the effect may be related to insulin sensitizing effect or the associated weight loss. Pioglitazone has not been shown to have any effect. Melatonin given at a dose of 2 mg for 6 months has been shown to reduce testosterone levels. However, benefit on sleep parameters is yet to be defined.

Modafinil and Armodafinil have been used as wake promoting drugs in patients who have residual sleepiness despite the regular use of CPAP. However, it should not be given to patients wishing to conceive and if given in child-bearing age, adequate contraception should be advised. Solriamfetol is another drug, which is a dopamine, norepinephrine reuptake inhibitor (DNRI) that can be used to treat excessive daytime sleepiness due to OSA.

Research gap:

1. Type I to IV sleep studies and applicability in PCOS group needs further studied.
2. There is need for ongoing trials that look specifically at larger groups of OSA in PCOS country wise and assess if CPAP therapy has any beneficial impact on the reproductive health and metabolic parameters in PCOS.

5.5.4. How to evaluate and treat Insomnia in PCOS?

Draft recommendations:

5.5.4.1. Chronic insomnia in PCOS needs to be teased out further to see whether it is an independent association or part of the mood disturbances that is very common in PCOS. *(High quality of evidence)*

5.5.4.2. Insomnia should be effectively treated to improve quality of life. *(High quality of evidence)*

Summary of evidence: Chronic insomnia is defined as inability to fall asleep and difficulty in getting back to sleep once awake in the night (sleep-onset and sleep maintenance insomnia respectively), that lasts at least 3 nights a week for ≥3 months.

Treating underlying mood disorders and stress management will be essential. When symptoms persist Z drugs (nonbenzodiazepines such as zolpidem and zopiclone) can be tried and generally not for >4 weeks. Nonpharmacological therapy such as cognitive behavioral therapy (CBT), relaxation and multicomponent therapy, sleep hygiene instructions help to alleviate symptoms to a great extent.[10]

Research gap:

1. CBT for insomnia in PCOS needs further studies in larger groups to know the long-term impact.

5.5.5. What is the management of Restless legs (RLS, Willis-Ekbom Disease) in PCOS?

Draft recommendations:

5.5.5.1. PCOS patients should be specifically asked for restless legs when sleep health is being evaluated. *(Low quality of evidence)*

Summary of evidence: In small sample size studies, it has been shown that RLS is common in PCOS than the normal controls. RLS is normally reported by 5–15% of the general population. It can be either idiopathic or secondary to iron deficiency (low ferritin levels), chronic kidney disease, diabetes mellitus, peripheral neuropathy or drugs (antidepressants such as venlafaxine, dopamine antagonists and occasionally antihistamines). It is an under diagnosed and undertreated condition even in the general population with significant impact on the physical and mental health of the affected patients.

It is a condition where there is intense urge to move the lower limbs usually toward evenings or at rest and there is relief on walking or moving the legs. Associated paresthesia may be present. Type I PSG monitoring the leg electromyogram (EMG) will be required to demonstrate the periodic limb movements to confirm the diagnosis. Movements are 5–10 seconds long, separated by 4–90 seconds and in a sequence of at least four movements with

EMG elevation of 8 microvolts. Not all with periodic limb movements on PSG have RLS.

Supplementing iron even when ferritin is in the normal range can help. Dopamine agonists such as ropinirole and pramipexole are well tolerated and effective for symptomatic RLS. Nonpharmacological therapies such as reflexology, stretching exercises, and massage therapy have all been tried with variable benefits but with significant alleviation of symptoms in chronic kidney disease patients.

Research gap:

1. The effect of RLS on cardiometabolic status and daytime functioning needs further studies in PCOS.

CONCLUSION

1. Sleep health assessment should be an integral part of evaluation of PCOS.
2. In those who are symptomatic of underlying sleep disorders, appropriate sleep study should be carried out after a formal clinical evaluation. In those with high clinical probability of sleep apnea with no other suspected sleep disorders, a portable home study (type III) will suffice. When there are uncommon features, restless legs, etc., technician led, lab-based type I polysomnography remains the gold standard.
3. Lifestyle modifications, sleep hygiene, dietary interventions are important aspects. For those with symptomatic OSA, CPAP should be given, not only to improve daytime symptoms but also for the likely reduction in cardiometabolic adverse effects. In patients intolerant of CPAP and symptomatic, mandibular advancement device is an option.
4. Close collaboration of the gynecologist with sleep physician, psychiatrist, dentist, ENT and nutritionist will be mandatory for comprehensive care delivery to improve outcome in this challenging PCOS patients.

REFERENCES

1. Teede H, Tassone EC, Piltonen T, et al. Effect of the combined oral contraceptive pill and/or metformin in the management of polycystic ovary syndrome: a systematic review with meta-analyses. Clin Endocrinol (Oxf). 2019;91:479-89.
2. Hachul H, Polesel DN, Tock L, Sleep disorders in polycystic ovary syndrome: influence of obesity and hyperandrogenism. Reva Assoc Med Bras. 1992;65(3):375-83.
3. Kumarendran B, Sumilo D, O'Reilly MW, et al. Increased risk of obstructive sleep apnoea in women with polycystic ovary syndrome: a population-based cohort study. Eur J Endocrinol. 2019;180(4):265-72.
4. Nagappa M, Liao P, Wong J, et al. Validation of the STOP-Bang Questionnaire as a screening tool for obstructive sleep apnea among different populations: a systematic review and meta-analysis. PLoS One. 2015;10(12):e0143697.

5. Kapur VK, Auckley DH, Chowdhuri S, et al. Clinical practice guideline for diagnostic testing for adult obstructive sleep apnea: an American Academy of Sleep Medicine clinical practice guideline. J Clin Sleep Med. 2017;13(3):479-504.
6. American Academy of Sleep Medicine. AASM Manual for the Scoring of Sleep and Associated Events: Rules, Terminology and Technical Specifications. Darien, IL: American Academy of Sleep Medicine; 2023.
7. Wong AM, Barnes HN, Joosten SA, et al. The effect of surgical weight loss on obstructive sleep apnoea: a systematic review and meta-analysis. Sleep Med Rev. 2018;42:85-99.
8. Rueda JR, Mugueta-Aguinaga I, Vilaró J, et al. Myofunctional therapy (oropharyngeal exercises) for obstructive sleep apnoea. Cochrane Database Syst Rev. 2020;11:CD013449.
9. Liu A, Kim SH, Ariel D, et al. Does enhanced insulin sensitivity improve sleep measures in patients with obstructive sleep apnea: a randomized, placebo-controlled pilot study. Sleep Med. 2016;22:57-60.
10. Demir Çaltekin M, Hamamci M, Onat T, et al. Evaluation of sleep quality, restless legs syndrome, anxiety and depression in polycystic ovary syndrome. J Turk Sleep Med. 2021;8(3):243-9.

CHAPTER 6

Screening and Management for Infertility till Intrauterine Insemination

Sonia Malik, Aneesha Grover

INTRODUCTION

Polycystic ovarian syndrome (PCOS) is an enigmatic disorder having many phenotypes and resultant dysfunctions. Infertility forms a major symptom of the disorder and ovulatory dysfunction forms the major cause for infertility in these patients. Most treatments aim at either inducing or augmenting ovulation in order to treat infertility. The treatment is varied because of the varied phenotypic presentations of these anovulatory patients. All grades of management regimens from simple like ovulation induction and timed intercourse to complex and advanced treatments like IUI and IVF are found in literature. It becomes imperative therefore to collate evidence-based recommendations so that they can be applied to the various patients according to their requirement. Intrauterine insemination (IUI) is a simple technique that has been popularly used for decades in various types of infertility. The anovulatory PCOS patient is offered simple OI and timed intercourse as the first-line treatment. If unsuccessful, IUI is offered as a second step, and finally she may undergo laparoscopic ovarian drilling or IVF if there are IUI failures as well.

6.1. What are the preconception risk factors associated with poor or negative fertility outcomes?

Draft recommendations:

6.1.1. The preconception risk factors associated with poor or negative fertility outcomes are: *(Low quality of evidence)*

- i. Maternal age >35 years
- ii. Obesity with BMI >30 kg/m^2
- iii. *Number of cycles:* >3 previous cycles of IUI
- iv. *Type of infertility:* Primary infertility
- v. Duration of infertility of >4.8 years

6.1.2. In PCOS women planning for pregnancy it is important to evaluate weight, blood pressure, lipid profile, lifestyle including addictions, nutrition, exercise, and sleep. *(Low quality of evidence)*

6.1.3. One should optimize the reproductive outcome by healthy lifestyle, prevention of excess weight gain, and optimizing preconception risk factors, mental, emotional, and sexual health. *(Clinical practice point)*

6.1.4. Chronic conditions such as diabetes, high blood pressure, anxiety, depression, and other mental health conditions should be optimally managed and women should be counseled regarding the risk of adverse pregnancy outcomes. *(Clinical practice point)*

Summary of evidence: Lifestyle modification is the first-line treatment for PCOS and a loss of even 5–10% of the bodyweight in overweight and obese PCOS patients is beneficial to the improvement of their reproductive and metabolic parameters. The changes in the implantation rate, pregnancy rate, and live birthrate by age were significantly slower for PCOS patients than for non-PCOS patients. Kalra et al. (2013) found that in spite of higher number of oocytes being retrieved in each age group of PCOS women, the pregnancy rates and live birthrates for that age did not change when compared to non-PCOS women.[1] The excess androgen in PCOS results in central obesity which increases the insulin resistance. This, in turn, results in more hyperandrogenemia resulting in dysfunction of the H-P-O axis, anovulation, and infertility. Women with PCO trying to achieve a pregnancy should keep their BMI between 19 and 29 kg/m^2. Guan et al. (2022), however, did not find any significant difference in the rates of clinical pregnancies, miscarriage, ectopic pregnancies, live births, multiple pregnancies, or the delivery method in the different BMI groups.[2] According to the International Evidence based guidelines (2023), compared to overweight and obese PCO, the lean and normal weight PCO women have a better pregnancy rate and live birthrate.[3]

In PCOS women undergoing IUI, the cumulative CPR and LBR increase as the number of cycles increases up to the third cycle and then plateaus thereafter.[2] Type of infertility and duration of infertility also influenced the pregnancy rates in PCOS women treated by ovulation induction with timed intercourse or IUI. The CPR in primary infertility group was significantly lower than the secondary infertility group.[2] Longer the duration of infertility, lower is the probability of conception, especially if it exceeds 4.8 years.[4] The live birthrates in women undergoing IUI was higher in those with a shorter duration of infertility (3.5 ± 2.1 years vs. 4.7 ± 3.9 years).[4]

Research gap: There are no studies that implicate the metabolic features of PCOS as a direct cause of decreased fecundity. The impact of duration of infertility on pregnancy rates is not clear.

6.2. Is it necessary to confirm that patient is anovulatory before starting any treatment?

Draft recommendation:

6.2.1. Since OI cycles are associated with better results than natural cycles irrespective of ovulatory status of the woman, confirmation of anovulation before starting treatment is not necessary. *(Low quality of evidence)*

Summary of evidence: About 15% of patients with infertility present with ovulatory dysfunction out of which 80% of these are related to PCOS.

When natural cycle IUI was compared with IUI following ovulation induction, the pregnancy rates were significantly higher in older (38–40 years) women undergoing OI-IUI versus natural cycle IUI in that age group.[5] However, in younger women the pregnancy rate was similar in both the groups. In another study by Li et al. (2020), it was seen that even in women with regular menstrual cycles, OI with gonadotropins followed by IUI gave better results than natural cycle IUI.[6]

Research gap: There is paucity of evidence in describing the tests that are mandatory before starting an OI cycle in PCOS. There is a controversy on whether day 2 hormonal tests should be done or not in these patients once the diagnosis of PCOS is confirmed.

6.3. What test would you do before inducing ovulation?

Draft recommendations:

6.3.1. To diagnose PCOS one must exclude other disorders with following tests. *(Low quality of evidence)*

Pregnancy	***Beta-hCG***
Ovarian failure	FSH
Hypothyroidism	TSH
Hyperprolactinemia	Prolactin
CAH	17-OH progesterone
Ovarian tumor	Total testosterone (especially if >200 ng/dL)
Adrenal tumor	DHEAS (especially if >800 µg/dL)
Cushing syndrome	Serum cortisol

6.3.2. In women with PCOS and infertility due to anovulation alone with normal semen analysis, the risks, benefits, costs, and timing and techniques of tubal patency testing in relation to the cost and complexity of the treatment should be considered on an individual basis, depending on personal history and population prevalence, prior to starting ovulation induction with timed intercourse or intrauterine insemination. *(Moderate quality of evidence)*

6.3.3. Free androgen index by testing total testosterone and SHBG may be necessary in the absence of clinical hyperandrogenemia. *(Moderate quality of evidence)*

6.3.4. Baseline ultrasound to rule out any other pelvic abnormality and for estimating the AFC. *(Low quality of evidence)*

6.3.5. Testing for impaired glucose tolerance, lipid profile, and metabolic disorders is essential. *(Moderate quality of evidence)*

Summary of evidence: Few basic investigations to rule out contraindications to ovulation induction are necessary. These include a semen analysis and tubal patency testing by HSG or sonosalpingography. There is not much evidence to suggest that PCOS is associated with tubal pathology. The uterine pathologies can be identified by the baseline ultrasound done in all patients before staring medication for ovulation Induction.[7]

Research gaps: It is still controversial whether tubal patency testing in necessary in all PCOS women before ovulation induction. It is suggested that it may be necessary only in those patients who are at a higher risk of tubal abnormalities with history of previous abdominal septic surgery like peritonitis or pelvic surgical procedures, sexual transmitted infection, or pelvic inflammatory disease or a positive serum test for sexually transmitted infection and presence of concomitant endometriosis.

6.4. Which oral ovulogens will you use and why?

Draft recommendations:

6.4.1. Letrozole should be the first-line pharmacological treatment for ovulation induction in infertile anovulatory women with PCOS, with no other infertility factors. *(High quality of evidence)*

6.4.2. The use of letrozole is still off-label in many countries, where it is not allowed, clinicians should use other ovulation induction agents. *(Clinical practice point)*

6.4.3. Clomiphene citrate could be used as a second-line pharmacological treatment for ovulation induction. *(Moderate quality of evidence)*

6.4.4. Metformin could be used alone, in women with PCOS with anovulatory infertility and, to improve clinical pregnancy and live birthrates, after informing women that there are more effective ovulation agents. *(High quality of evidence)*

6.4.5. Clomiphene citrate combined with metformin could be used rather than clomiphene citrate or metformin alone in women with PCOS with anovulatory infertility to improve ovulation and clinical pregnancy rates. *(Moderate quality of evidence)*

6.4.6. Current evidence demonstrates no difference in fetal abnormality rates between letrozole and/or clomiphene citrate ovulation induction or natural conception. *(Clinical practice point)*

Summary of evidence: Clomiphene citrate and letrozole for ovulation induction followed with IUI is superior to expectant management and natural-cycle IUI. Many studies have been conducted to compare the efficacy of various ovulogens for OI in women with PCOS. Letrozole was superior to clomiphene citrate for ovulation rate (per patient and per cycle); pregnancy rate, clinical pregnancy rate and live birthrate per patient.[3,8-10]

There were no differences between letrozole and clomiphene citrate for other outcomes including multiple pregnancy rate (per patient or pregnancy); and miscarriage rate (per patient or pregnancy).[3,8-10]

Addition of metformin was beneficial when combined with clomiphene citrate rather than letrozole.[3,10] Gonadotrophins were superior for live birthrate, clinical pregnancy rate per patient, and ovulation rate per cycle but may be associated with multiple pregnancies and ovarian hyperstimulation syndrome (OHSS) if conventional protocols used.[3,10]

Research gap: There is no analysis on the usage of drugs based on the phenotype of the patient, hence OI lacks individualization.

Despite the benefit being demonstrated for use of letrozole with no increase in congenital anomalies, there is lack of approval by regulatory agencies, in certain countries. This may limit implementation of the international guidelines 2023 and should be revisited in light of the evidence and recommendations presented.[3]

6.5. How will you manage resistance to oral ovulogens?

Draft recommendations:

6.5.1. Lifestyle modification with diet and exercise to keep BMI between 19 and 30 kg/m^2 is recommended. But, one must take into consideration the age of the patient as with increasing age the chance of conception decreases. *(High quality of evidence)*

6.5.2. Addition of metformin may be beneficial when combined with clomiphene citrate to induce ovulation in addition to correcting hyperinsulinemia. *(Moderate quality of evidence)*

6.5.3. Glucocorticoids may be given in resistant cases. *(Low quality of evidence)*

6.5.4. Alternative options for OI in case of resistance include: *(Low quality of evidence)*
   a. Extended therapy of letrozole and clomiphene citrate
   b. Change the oral ovulogen
   c. Combination of Letrozole and clomiphene citrate

6.5.5. Gonadotropins could be second-line pharmacological therapy for women with PCOS who are anovulatory with oral ovulogens. Gonadotrophins could be used alone or in combination with letrozole and clomiphene citrate. *(Moderate quality of evidence)*

6.5.6. Laparoscopic ovarian drilling (LOD) could be second-line therapy for women with PCOS who are anovulatory and infertile, with clomiphene citrate resistance. *(Moderate quality of evidence)*

6.5.7. IVF could be offered in women with PCOS and anovulatory infertility, if first- or second-line ovulation induction therapies have failed. *(Moderate quality of evidence)*

Summary of evidence: Major factors that contribute toward resistance to OI are obesity, insulin resistance, and hyperandrogenemia. Lifestyle modification, which includes diet, exercise, de-addiction, and adequate sleep forms an essential part of the management for resistance to oral ovulogens. Even 5–10% of weight loss can reduce central fat by up to 30% and improve insulin sensitivity and reduce insulin resistance. It restores ovulation and increases fertility along with other health benefits on metabolic symptoms. It may reduce the occurrence of miscarriage rate and gestational diabetes. Metformin when used in combination with clomiphene citrate is known to improve the ovulation and clinical pregnancy rate but not increase the livebirth rate.[3]

There is some evidence for extended clomiphene or letrozole therapy. The use of letrozole or extended treatment with clomiphene did not increase ovulation rates, and occurrence of pregnancy, and improve pregnancy outcomes.[11] Statistically superior effect of the extended letrozole regimen over a conventional regimen was not detected.[12] Combination of letrozole and CC was associated with a higher ovulation rate compared with letrozole alone.[13] Further studies are needed to evaluate the effect on LBR. Use of dexamethasone plus CC in CC resistant women with elevated DHEAS levels has been supported by a few studies.[14]

Livebirth rate, clinical pregnancy rate per patient, and ovulation rate per cycle are higher with gonadotrophins than with clomiphene citrate though the incidence of multiple pregnancies and OHSS is higher.[3] There was some suggestion that in PCOS women gonadotropin can be used as the first line of treatment for ovulation induction. More studies are required to establish gonadotropins as first-line treatment in IUI cycles in order to improve pregnancy rates. When gonadotropins are prescribed, the cost of the intervention for ovulation induction, expertise required for the use of the intervention should be taken into consideration and stringent monitoring required. A low dose step-up gonadotropin protocol should be used to optimize the chance of monofollicular development and prevent complications.

LOD destroys ovarian androgen-producing tissue with fall in the serum levels of androgens, LH, and inhibin followed by increase in FSH levels. Both local and systemic effects promote follicular recruitment, growth, maturation, and subsequent ovulation, and are able to restore CC sensitivity and prevent OHSS.[15]

When using laparoscopic ovarian surgery, the following should be considered:

a. Comparative cost of the intervention for ovulation induction.
b. Expertise required for the safe use of the intervention for ovulation induction.
c. Both intraoperative and postoperative risks, which are higher in women who are obese.

When FSH is compared to LOD, FSH was found to be superior to LOD for live birthrates, but higher rates of multiple pregnancies per patient were significant.[15] Therefore, informed shared decision-making can allow choice of second-line therapy based on patient preferences and priorities.

Research gap: The evidence for alternative oral therapies, combination therapies, and lifestyle modification are of very low quality. One needs to weigh its benefit as compared to gonadotropin therapy. Additional prospective trials with larger sample sizes are needed to assess the ovulatory effects of these regimens. Gonadotropin therapy requires adequate resource (trained medical/nursing personnel and ultrasound machinery), specialist access, and monitoring. Moreover gonadotropin preparations are significantly more expensive than oral agents and require parenteral administration and close monitoring with regular ultrasound with a higher risk of multiple pregnancy compared with oral agents or surgery.

Though LOD is efficacious, single procedure, requiring no monitoring, and additional costs for ovulation indiuction, there is high risk of adhesion formation and decreased ovarian reserve.

CONCLUSION

Management of infertility in PCOS patients is an art that needs fine-tuning. There is a high possibility of under stimulation because of the risk of multiple pregnancies and OHSS. The patient therefore needs to be handled very carefully so that she can be optimally stimulated—neither low nor excessive. Medications must be well known to the physician to gauge what is best suited for the patient in question. A treatment algorithm must be made and followed properly and diligently to get best result. One needs to balance the benefits with the evidence when using alternative treatments in women resistant to oral ovulogens.

REFERENCES

1. Kalra SK, Ratcliffe SJ, Dokras A. Is the fertile window extended in women with polycystic ovary syndrome? Utilizing the Society for Assisted Reproductive Technology registry to assess the impact of reproductive aging on live-birth rate. Fertil Steril. 2013;100(1):208-13.
2. Guan HJ, Pan LQ, Song H, et al. Predictors of pregnancy after intrauterine insemination in women with polycystic ovary syndrome. J Int Med Res. 2021;49(5):3000605211018600.
3. Teede HJ, Tay CT, Laven JJ, et al. Recommendations from the 2023 international evidence-based guideline for the assessment and management of polycystic ovary syndrome. Eur J Endocrinol. 2023;189(2):G43-64.
4. Pekcan KM, Tokmak A, Ulubasoglu H, et al. The importance of infertility duration and follicle size according to pregnancy success in women undergoing

ovulation induction with gonadotropins and intrauterine insemination. J Obstet Gynaecol. 2023;43(1):2173058.
5. Richter KS, Yamasaki MM, Hill J, et al. Natural Cycle Intrauterine Insemination (IUI) versus Ovulation Induction (OI) for Non-Infertile women. Fertil Steril Oral Session. 2018;110(Suppl 4):e20-1.
6. Li S, He Y, Cao M, Liu H, et al. Low-dose human menopausal gonadotrophin versus natural cycles in intrauterine insemination for subfertile couples with regular menstruation. J Ovarian Res. 2020;13(1):36.
7. Legro RS, Brzyski RG, Diamond MP, et al. Letrozole versus clomiphene for infertility in the polycystic ovary syndrome. N Engl J Med. 2014;371:119-29.
8. Tsiami AP, Goulis DG, Sotiriadis AI, et al. Higher ovulation rate with letrozole as compared with clomiphene citrate in infertile women with polycystic ovary syndrome: a systematic review and meta-analysis. Hormones (Athens). 2021;20(3):449-61.
9. Wang B, Li Z. Hypersecretion of basal luteinizing hormone and an increased risk of pregnancy loss among women with polycystic ovary syndrome undergoing controlled ovarian stimulation and intrauterine insemination. Heliyon. 2023;9(5):e16233.
10. Franik S, Eltrop SM, Kremer JA, et al. Aromatase inhibitors (letrozole) for subfertile women with polycystic ovary syndrome. Cochrane Database Syst Rev. 2018;5(5):CD010287. Update in: Cochrane Database Syst Rev. 2022;9: CD010287.
11. Emara MA, Mohamed DI, Hassanein MA, et al. Letrozole therapy versus extended clomiphene citrate therapy for induction of ovulation in resistant patients with polycystic ovarian syndrome in low resource communities. Egyptian J Hospital Med. 2020;81(7):2456-61.
12. Zhu X, Lang J, Wang Q, et al. Extended versus conventional letrozole regimen in patients with polycystic ovary syndrome undergoing their first ovulation induction cycle: a prospective randomized controlled trial. Hum Reprod Open. 2024;2024(3):hoae046.
13. Mejia RB, Summers KM, Kresowik JD, et al. A randomized controlled trial of combination letrozole and clomiphene citrate or letrozole alone for ovulation induction in women with polycystic ovary syndrome. Fertil Steril. 2019;111(3):571-8.
14. Thabet M, Abdelrazik MM. Adding prednisolone during ovulation induction with clomiphene citrate in lean women with clomiphene citrate resistant polycystic ovarian syndrome. Egyptian J Fertil Steril. 2019;23(1):16-22.
15. Farquhar C, Brown J, Marjoribanks J. Laparoscopic drilling by diathermy or laser for ovulation induction in anovulatory polycystic ovary syndrome. Cochrane Database Syst Rev. 2012;6:CD001122.

CHAPTER 7

Role of ART in PCOS: Increasing Efficiency and Reducing Complications

N Sanjeeva Reddy, Radha Vembu

INTRODUCTION

PCOS is a common endocrine disorder among women of the reproductive age group. PCOS women with anovulatory infertility, IVF/ICSI is recommended when there is resistance or failure with first- or second-line ovulation induction treatment or for those who require IVF for other indications or have a high response gonadotropin cycle. There could be several challenges during ovarian stimulation (OS), like the risk of ovarian hyperstimulation syndrome (OHSS), high serum estradiol levels, embryo-endometrial asynchrony, and the need for freeze all strategy.

7.1. What are the indications for ART in women with PCOS?

Draft recommendation:

7.1.1. In PCOS women with anovulatory infertility, IVF/ICSI is recommended when first- or second-line ovulation induction treatment have failed[1] or in the presence of absolute indication like tubal factor, male factor, severe endometriosis, low ovarian reserve or when PGT is required to prevent aneuploidy and genetically inherited disease. *(Low quality of evidence)*

Summary of evidence: The current evidence supports letrozole as the first-line treatment for ovulation induction. If conception does not occur with oral ovulogens, gonadotropins are considered as the second-line treatment. However, if the patient cannot afford gonadotropins or if follicular monitoring is not feasible, laparoscopic ovarian drilling (LOD) can be considered. If conception still does not occur, assisted reproductive technology (ART) is considered the third-line treatment. Additionally, maternal age is a crucial predictor of the treatment outcome. Moreover, ART is also indicated if the patient fails to conceive after 3 to 6 cycles of ovulation induction followed by intrauterine insemination or has any other indication that requires ART.

Research gap: There is no clear evidence suggesting when to proceed with ART and after how many unsuccessful IUI cycles. Further research is required on deciding for ART as first-line treatment based on other prognostic factors such as age, previous ovarian surgeries, patient choice, time to conception, and cost. One must also take into consideration the higher risk of ovarian hyperstimulation syndrome, multiple pregnancies, and miscarriage.

7.2. What is the COS protocol of choice?

Draft recommendations:

7.2.1. The antagonist protocol is recommended as it allows the use of GnRH agonist trigger with the freezing of all embryos generated, if required, without compromising the cumulative live birth rate, to reduce the risk of ovarian hyperstimulation syndrome (OHSS). *(High quality of evidence)*.

7.2.2. There is insufficient evidence to recommend a particular type of gonadotropin preparation. Either urinary or recombinant follicle stimulating hormone (FSH) or human menopausal hormone (hMG) could be used in women with PCOS undergoing controlled ovarian hyperstimulation for IVF/ICSI. *(Very low quality of evidence)*

Summary of evidence: The human chorionic gonadotropin (hCG), typically used to trigger ovulation, is often the primary cause of OHSS. The aim of a stimulation protocol in PCOS women will be synchronous follicular development with optimum oocyte maturation. The GnRH agonist protocol provides the benefit of improved oocyte yield and pregnancy rate but there is a sixfold increase in the risk of OHSS. This can be attributed to prolonged duration of stimulation and increased dose of gonadotropin requirement for OS. The agonist may prevent atresia of smaller follicles and allows to develop following down regulation, low basal FSH level may be sufficient to support the growth of multiple small follicles which in turn leads to more of intermediate follicles and increased risk of OHSS.[3,4] So, antagonist protocol is preferred over the agonist protocol for COS in PCOS women when there is concern of OHSS. There is no difference in the clinical pregnancy rates and live birth rates between the GnRH agonist and antagonist protocols.[2] [*Moderate quality of evidence* (OR 1.02 95% CI 0.85–1.23)]. But there is a significant reduction in the risk of OHSS (OR 0.61, 95% CI 0.51–0.72) and cycle cancellation for hyper- response (OR 0.47 95% CI 0.32–0.69).

There was no difference in the livebirth rates, safety or ovarian hyperstimulation syndrome rate irrespective of the gonadotropin used.[1] Therefore the clinical choice of gonadotropin should depend on availability, convenience and costs of recombinant versus urinary and FSH versus hMG. There is insufficient evidence to determine the benefits of using or not using exogenous LH.[1]

Evidence gap: There is limited research on the other stimulation protocols in PCOS women like PPOS protocol and minimal stimulation. Further randomized control trials comparing newer protocols with antagonist protocol are required.

7.3. How will you prevent OHSS in women with PCOS?

Draft recommendations:

7.3.1. It is recommended to proceed with antagonist protocol to reduce the risk of moderate and severe OHSS in high responders or high-serum estradiol levels. *(High quality of evidence)*

7.3.2. As a first line strategy, it is recommended to use GnRH agonist as trigger for oocyte maturation to reduce the risk of OHSS. *(High quality of evidence)*

7.3.3. It is recommended for freeze all strategy and subsequent frozen embryo transfer to reduce the risk for early and late onset OHSS. *(High quality of evidence)*

7.3.4. It is recommended to individualize the dose of gonadotropins based on the ovarian reserve tests. *(Moderate quality of evidence)*

7.3.5. The risk of OHSS is increased when there are more than 17–19 mature follicles and elevated serum estradiol levels on the day of the trigger (greater than 3,500–5,000 pg/mL), as well as when more than 15–18 oocytes are retrieved. *(High quality of evidence)*

7.3.6. In patients at risk for moderate-to-severe OHSS, it is recommended to start cabergoline on the day of trigger or soon thereafter and continue for several days. Usually, it is administered in the dose of 0.5 mg once daily for 8 days. *(High quality of evidence)*

7.3.7. It is not recommended to use low dose of hCG only as trigger to reduce the risk of OHSS. *(Low quality of evidence)*

7.3.8. It is not recommended to administer letrozole to reduce the risk of moderate or severe OHSS as an intervention. *(Moderate quality of evidence)*

7.3.9. Volume expanders such as albumin, hydroxyethyl starch, and mannitol are not recommended as a preventive strategy for moderate or severe PCOS. *(Low quality of evidence)*

7.3.10. There is no recommendation to use Aspirin, mifepristone, myoinositol, D-chiro-inositol, or glucocorticoids to reduce OHSS risk. *(Low quality of evidence)*

7.3.11. The administration of a GnRH antagonist in the luteal phase is proposed to accelerate luteolysis, reduces ovarian VEGF secretion, and promotes the regression of OHSS symptoms. However, the evidence does not support the use of a GnRH antagonist alone postretrieval to reduce the risk of moderate to severe OHSS. *(Low quality of evidence)*

7.3.12. Coasting is not recommended as a primary strategy to reduce the risk of OHSS. However, it can be considered alongside other strategies, such as cabergoline and the freeze-all strategy, if more effective options are unavailable. *(Low quality of evidence)*

Summary of evidence: The preventive strategies should be considered in patients at risk of developing OHSS by using low risk treatment protocols and specific measures in individual cases. The parameters considered are as follows:

a. *Before the start of OS:* In women with elevated AMH (>3.4 ng/mL) and antral follicle count >24, young age, low BMI, hyper response to OS previously, anticipated high oocyte yield.
b. *Stimulation protocol:* In a Cochrane systemic review and meta-analysis, including 73 RCTs and 12,212 participants, there was statistically significant reduction in all the grades of OHSS (OR 0.61, 95% CI 0.51–0.72) with the antagonist protocol when compared to agonist protocol without significant reduction in LBR and increase in miscarriage rate.[2] A low dose gonadotropin protocol should be used during controlled ovarian stimulation.
c. *Ovulation trigger:* In an RCT of 66 women at high risk of OHSS, they compared GnRH agonist trigger and hCG trigger. There were no patients with OHSS in the agonist trigger group when compared to 31% of patients having OHSS in hCG trigger group.[5]
d. *Other drugs:* There is increased vascular permeability following release of vasoactive mediators from the stimulated ovaries. It is well known that vascular endothelial growth factor (VEGF) is a key mediator for OHSS. This VEGF forms an integral part of follicular growth, corpus luteal function, angiogenesis and vascular endothelial stimulation. In the presence of hCG, VEGF mediates vascular permeability of OHSS. Cabergoline reduces the effects of VEGF-mediated vascular permeability without compromising IR and PR *and is given in the dose* of 0.5 mg daily from day of hCG trigger for 7–10 days.[1] There is also some evidence for using IV calcium infusion (10 mL of 10% calcium gluconate in 200 mL normal saline) on the day of oocyte retrieval and thereafter on days 1, 2, and 3 after oocyte retrieval to decrease OHSS risk. There is not much evidence for other adjuvant therapies.

Evidence gap: There is limited research on the role of continuation of GnRH antagonist postoocyte retrieval or use of letrozole to keep estradiol levels low in patients at risk of OHSS, which is a feasible option in low-resource settings and this warrants larger studies.

7.4. How will you manage OHSS?

Draft recommendations (RCOG guideline 5):[6]

7.4.1. Outpatient management is considered in patients with mild or moderate OHSS and selected cases of severe OHSS. *(Very low quality of evidence)*

7.4.2. Women undergoing outpatient management of OHSS should be counseled regarding fluid intake and output monitoring and they should be provided with contact details to access advice. *(Very low quality of evidence)*

7.4.3. Nonsteroidal anti-inflammatory agents should be avoided, as they may compromise renal function. *(Very low quality of evidence)*

7.4.4. Women with severe OHSS being managed on an outpatient basis should receive thromboprophylaxis with LMWH. The duration of treatment should be individualized, based on risk factors and whether conception occurs or not. *(Very low quality of evidence)*

7.4.5. Paracentesis of ascitic fluid may be carried out on an outpatient basis by the abdominal or transvaginal route under ultrasound guidance. *(Very low quality of evidence)*

7.4.6. There is insufficient evidence to support the use of GnRH antagonists or dopamine agonists in treating established cases of OHSS. *(Very low quality of evidence)*

Summary of evidence: OHSS is self-limiting and resolution parallels decrease in serum hCG levels. It usually occurs within 7 days in nonpregnant women and takes about 10–20 days in pregnant women. Mild and moderate OHSS can be treated on OPD basis but moderate OHSS requires more frequent evaluation and monitoring. Severe cases need hospitalization and stringent monitoring, which is mainly supportive with multidisciplinary management protocols involving gynecologists, anesthetists, hematologists and intensivist. Management involves circulatory support using IV fluids, maintenance of renal function, thromboprophylaxis and drainage of third space accumulation in case of dyspnea or tachypnea. Counseling regarding the signs and symptoms of progressing illness is necessary. Daily communication, to ensure that progression to more severe disease is promptly recognized. Frequent evaluation by physical and USG examinations, daily weight and urine output measurements along with serial laboratory determinations of hematocrit, electrolytes, and serum creatinine is necessary.

Fluid management: These women should be counseled regarding monitoring of fluid intake and output. They should be encouraged to take fluid to thirst rather than a fixed amount.[6]

Drugs: Nonsteroidal anti-inflammatory agents should be avoided as they can compromise renal function. GnRH antagonist at 250 μg/day for 3–5 days, combined with the continued use of a dopamine agonist like cabergoline, may lead to quicker regression of clinical features in established cases of early OHSS.

Inpatient management: Women with OHSS should be admitted when they are:

- Unable to achieve pain control with outpatient management
- Unable to have adequate fluid intake due to nausea.
- Worsening of clinical features of OHSS in spite of outpatient care
- Unable to have regular outpatient follow-up
- Having critical OHSS

Patients with critical OHSS and severe OHSS with persistent hemoconcentration and dehydration require multidisciplinary team approach and intensive care. In majority of cases, crystalloids are useful for initial correction of dehydration. However, colloids are preferred like human albumin and hexaethyl starch (HES) for correction of dehydration in severe OHSS. Those women with persistent hemoconcentration in spite of volume replacement with colloids need invasive monitoring in ICU setup.

Diuretics should be avoided as they deplete intravascular volume further except in situations where oliguria is persisting in spite of adequate fluid replacement and drainage of ascites.

Paracentesis is indicated in severe abdominal distension and abdominal pain secondary to ascites, shortness of breath and respiratory compromise, oliguria despite adequate volume replacement.

Thromboprophylaxis: LMWH thromboprophylaxis should be considered in women with severe or critical OHSS and those inpatients admitted for OHSS. The duration of prophylaxis should be individualized based on the risk factors and outcome of treatment.

Indications for surgical management: Surgery is indicated if there is associated adnexal torsion, ovarian rupture or ectopic pregnancy and it should be performed only by an experienced surgeon.

Evidence gap: As all these recommendations are based on smaller studies, case reports and expert opinion, there is lack of RCTs and meta-analysis.

7.5. Is in vitro maturation (IVM) of oocytes treatment of choice in women with PCOS?

Draft recommendations:

7.5.1. IVM should be considered only when there is sufficient expertise, as an option in women with prior severe OHSS and with increased risk in present stimulation, acknowledging the lower cumulative livebirth rate. *(Moderate quality of evidence)*

7.5.2. Evidence suggests that IVM/ICSI is less effective than standard IVF/ICSI in terms of clinical pregnancy and livebirth rate per patient. *(Clinical practice points)*

Summary of evidence: IVM is tried in women who are at high risk of OHSS as there is less requirement of medications for stimulation, with shorter duration of stimulation, less monitoring and financial burden. IVM refers to maturation of cumulus oocyte complexes in culture from germinal vesicle stage through meiosis I and then to reach metaphase II where the follicles are not exposed to preovulatory trigger. In IVM, a high level of attrition is observed from oocyte to blastocyst due to sub optimal nuclear and cytoplasmic maturation and so this area warrants more research. IVM may be combined with ICSI but vitrification of immature oocytes is not recommended due to poor outcomes.

So IVM provides an alternate treatment protocol in women with high risk for OHSS but they should be appropriately counseled about expected results and informed consent. It might be an option only in women with a high AFC and they should be informed about lower blastocyst conversion and that implantation and pregnancy rates may be reduced when compared to conventional IVF.[7]

Evidence gap: The potential for epigenetic disruptions like abnormal methylations of maternally expressed genes, needs careful evaluation of oocytes matured in vitro.

Information regarding safety of these children is limited regarding the malformation and developmental outcomes and this warrants long term studies with large sample size.

7.6. Should metformin be used in all patients undergoing ART?

Draft recommendations:

7.6.1. It is not recommended to give metformin for the sole purpose of reducing OHSS in PCOS women in GnRH antagonist cycles. However, it can be considered to reduce the risk of OHSS in women undergoing GnRH agonist protocol. *(Moderate quality of evidence)*

7.6.2. It can be considered in women with hirsutism, insulin resistance and central obesity. *(Very low quality of evidence)*

Summary of evidence: Metformin is an insulin sensitizer used in women with PCOS. It can affect the ovarian response by reducing the number of non-periovulatory follicles and hence the estradiol secretion. The administration of metformin during OS in GnRH agonist protocol decreased the incidence of OHSS in PCOS women and this is supported in a meta-analysis of 1,516 participants (RR 0.44 95% CI 0.26–0.77) compared to controls.[8]

In an RCT including 496 participants in GnRH antagonist protocol, there was no significant reduction in the incidence of moderate to severe OHSS with metformin when compared to controls (3.6% vs 7.5% $p = 0.421$).[9]

If metformin is used, the following points could be considered:

- Commence metformin at the start of GnRH agonist treatment and gradually titrate the dose till a dose of 1,000–2,500 mg per day is reached to minimize the side effects.
- Can stop metformin at the time of pregnancy test or periods unless metformin therapy is indicated.[10] *(Practice points)*

Evidence gap: Exposure to metformin and long-term outcome of the neonate is still uncertain and further studies are required.

7.7. How important is lifestyle modification in patients who need ART? What is the evidence?

Draft recommendations:

7.7.1. Lifestyle intervention (exercise alone or multicomponent diet combined with exercise and behavioral strategies) should be recommended for all women with PCOS, for improving metabolic health including central adiposity and lipid profile. *(High quality of evidence)*

7.7.2. Healthy lifestyle behavior includes healthy eating and/or physical activity and is recommended in all PCOS women to optimize general health, quality of life, body composition, and weight management. *(High quality of evidence)*

7.7.3. *Exercise intervention:* It is recommended to encourage these women to undertake physical activity. They should aim for a minimum of 150–300 minutes of moderate intensity activity or 75–150 minutes of vigorous intensity aerobic activity per week or combination of both spread throughout the week along with muscle strengthening activities on two nonconsecutive days per week. *(High quality of evidence)*

7.7.4. As per 2023, PCOS guidelines, there is no evidence to support one type of diet composition over the other. The diet composition should be consistent with the population guidelines and should advice healthy eating tailored to individual goals and preferences. *(Clinical practice point)*

Summary of evidence:

Dietary intervention: PCOS women tend to have insulin resistance and increase the risk of type II diabetes. So, life style modifications including dietary changes help in weight loss, reduce insulin resistance, incidence of type II diabetes, reduce hyperandrogenism and regularize the menstrual cycle and hence improves fertility. The diet should include fruits and vegetables low in glycemic index, usually non starchy, low-fat dairy, diet rich in polyunsaturated fatty acids. Along with diet, hydration, and exercise is required.

Exercise intervention: For more benefits with moderate weight loss and prevention of weight regain, they should aim for a minimum of 250 min/week of moderate intensity activity or 150 min/week of vigorous intensity activity or a combination of both in addition to muscle strengthening activities on at least two nonconsecutive days per week.

Evidence gap: Recognizing the importance of individualized interventions, identifying the knowledge gaps and improving the quality of life needs attention.

7.8. How to prevent complications in ART?

Draft recommendations:

7.8.1. To prevent the risk of developing OHSS, it is preferred to plan antagonist protocol with agonist trigger and freeze all strategy. *(High quality of evidence)*

7.8.2. If fresh embryo transfer is planned, one should opt for single embryo transfer to prevent occurrence of multiple pregnancy. *(High quality of evidence)*

Summary of evidence: PCOS women are at increased risk of OHSS. This can be prevented by individualized OS protocol, starting with low dose of gonadotropins, administration of agonist trigger for oocyte maturation, freeze all strategy, and plan for subsequent frozen embryo transfer.

Thrombotic complications can occur due to high estradiol levels in women with risk for OHSS which can be prevented by administrating low dose of gonadotropins, agonist trigger and adequate management of OHSS. The risk of multiple pregnancy can be reduced by single blastocyst transfer on Day 5.

Evidence gap: Further research on epigenetic modifications in embryos and its impact on long-term implications need to be addressed.

7.9. What is the role of freeze all in PCOS women undergoing ART?

Draft recommendation:

7.9.1. It is recommended to consider freeze all strategy and plan for frozen embryo transfer in a subsequent cycle in patients at risk for OHSS, with past history of OHSS with gonadotropin therapy and in those requiring PGT to rule out aneuploidy or single gene disorders. *(High quality of evidence)*

Summary of evidence: Elective freeze all strategy and transferring embryos in subsequent cycles can avoid the endogenous hCG rise with fresh embryo transfer cycles. This was a rescue strategy to prevent the OHSS. In a multicentric RCT of 2,157 patients, there was no significant difference in LBR between frozen and fresh embryo transfer cycles (48.7% vs. 50.2% respectively p = 0.50) but there was a significant reduction in incidence of moderate-to-severe OHSS.

In PCOS women with multifollicular development and with more intermediary follicles, GnRH agonist is given as a trigger instead of hCG trigger. This leads to reduction in steroidogenesis and early luteolysis. So the luteal phase will be defective and lowers the pregnancy rates with increase in miscarriage rates if fresh transfer is done with standard luteal support. Even if fresh transfer is planned, it requires intensive luteal support requiring small doses of hCG which can increase the risk of early OHSS and late OHSS with endogenous hCG. So freeze all strategy is followed in majority of patients.[11]

Evidence gap: Freeze all strategy is proven to be beneficial in PCOS women with respect to the risk of OHSS risk. But further research is essential to optimize the treatment protocols, outcome and more personalized reproductive care in these PCOS women as frozen embryo transfer may not be cost effective. There is limited data on long-term health outcomes in offsprings born out of frozen embryo transfer.

7.10. How will you prepare the endometrium for FET?

Draft recommendation:

7.10.1. Natural or stimulated cycle FET is preferred over HRT as the relaxin and other substances from the corpus luteum prevents the pregnancy complications like preeclampsia, diabetes mellitus, preterm labor, and intrauterine growth restriction. *(High quality of evidence)*

Summary of evidence: The choice of FET preparation in women with PCOS should be individualized, taking into account the patient's specific clinical scenario, cycle regularity, presence of ovulation, risk factors, and personal preferences. As most PCOS women have irregular or anovulatory cycles, FET can be done either in a stimulated or HRT cycle. In HRT cycles the medications have to be continued at least till placenta takes over the function (that is till 8–10 weeks of pregnancy). There is absence of corpus luteum which in turn leads to absence of relaxin and VEGF which affects the early placental development and increase the risk of hypertension during pregnancy.

The prolonged administration of exogenous estrogen increases the risk of thromboembolic events. This can be avoided by use of stimulated cycle FET with letrozole and or gonadotropins

In GnRH agonist pretreatment cycle, there is better control over the cycle and simplifies the synchronization between embryo and endometrial development in anovulatory and irregular cycle but not associated with improvement in live birth rate. Use of GnRH agonist decreases the cancellation rate and the need for more frequent USG and endocrine monitoring.[12] Moreover, the transfer time is more readily controlled. Despite its advantages, there are several disadvantages like increasing the duration of treatment and need for maintaining daily exogenous HRT throughout first trimester with increased risk of hypo estrogenic status and cyst formation.

In a cohort analysis, the LBR for natural cycle, stimulated cycle and HRT were 62.4%, 65.0%, and 52.2%, respectively. So stimulated cycle is preferred over natural cycle as many of these women have anovulatory cycles.[13]

Evidence gap: Further research is essential regarding the ideal protocol for endometrial preparation in FET cycles. Further personalized reproductive care is essential as frozen embryo transfer is the norm in PCOS women to avoid the risk of OHSS.

CONCLUSION

ART remains the third line of management for PCOS women. The clinicians should prefer an individualized OS protocol with careful monitoring to avoid the risk of OHSS. Also, antagonist protocol, agonist trigger, freeze all strategy and stimulated cycle FET with single blastocyst transfer can be a norm of choice to prevent complications and improve the ART outcome.

REFERENCES

1. Teede HJ, Tay CT, Laven JJ, et al. Recommendations from the 2023 international evidence-based guideline for the assessment and management of polycystic ovary syndrome. Eur J Endocrinol. 2023;189(2):G43-64.
2. Al-Inany HG, Youssef MA, Ayeleke R, et al. Gonadotrophin-releasing hormone antagonists for assisted reproductive technology. Cochrane Database Syst Rev. 2016;4:CD001750.
3. Practice Committee of the American Society for Reproductive Medicine. Prevention of moderate and severe ovarian hyperstimulation syndrome: a guideline. Fertil Steril. 2024;121:230-45.
4. Steward RG, Lan L, Shah AA, et al. Oocyte number as a predictor for ovarian hyperstimulation syndrome and live birth: an analysis of 256,381 in vitro fertilization cycles. Fertil Steril. 2014;101:967-73.
5. Engmann L, DiLuigi A, Schmidt D, et al. The use of gonadotropin–releasing hormone (GnRH) agonist to induce oocyte maturation after cotreatment with GnRH antagonist in high-risk patients undergoing in vitro fertilization prevents the risk of ovarian hyperstimulation syndrome: a prospective randomized controlled study. Fertil Steril. 2008;89:84-91.
6. Royal College of Obstetricians and Gynaecologists. The Management of Ovarian Hyperstimulation Syndrome (Green-top Guideline No. 5), 3rd edition. London: Royal College of Obstetricians and Gynaecologists; 2016.
7. Practice Committees of the American Society for Reproductive Medicine, the Society of Reproductive Biologists and Technologists, and the Society for Assisted Reproductive Technology. In vitro maturation: a committee opinion. Fertil Steril. 2021;115:298-304.
8. Huang X, Wang P, Tal R, et al. A systematic review and meta-analysis of metformin among patients with polycystic ovary syndrome undergoing assisted reproductive technology procedures. Int J Gynaecol Obstet. 2015;131:111-6.

9. Kalem MN, Kalem Z, Gurgan T. Effect of metformin and oral contraceptives on polycystic ovary syndrome and IVF cycles. J Endocrinol Invest. 2017;40:745-52.
10. European Society of Human Reproduction and Embryology. (2019). Guideline on Ovarian Stimulation for IVF/ICSI. [online] Available from https://www.eshre.eu/Guidelines-and-Legal/Guidelines/Ovarian-Stimulation-in-IVF-ICSI. [Last accessed November, 2024].
11. Lim SS, Hutchison SK, Van Ryswyk E, et al. Lifestyle changes in women with polycystic ovary syndrome. Cochrane Database Syst Rev. 2019;3(3):CD007506.
12. Ban M, Sun Y, Chen X, et al. Association between maternal polycystic ovarian syndrome undergoing assisted reproductive technology and pregnancy complications and neonatal outcomes: a systematic review and meta-analysis. J Ovarian Res. 2024;17:6.
13. Man Y, Bian Y, Zhao S, et al. The effect of different endometrial preparations on women with polycystic ovary syndrome undergoing initial frozen embryo transfer: a historical cohort analysis. Acta Obstet Gynecol Scand. 2021;100(6):1116-23.

8

CHAPTER

Pregnancy Outcome in Women with Polycystic Ovarian Syndrome

Sharmin Abbasi, Mohammad Noor-A-Alam

INTRODUCTION

There could be an adverse pregnancy outcome in women with polycystic ovarian syndrome (PCOS), and this is related to the presence of high BMI, metabolic disturbances, hyperandrogenism, and infertility.[1] The major cause of infertility is oligo-ovulation or anovulation, which requires ovulation induction or assisted reproductive technology (ART) to become pregnant. Evidence suggests that polycystic ovary syndrome has a negative impact on pregnancy outcomes, with an increased risk of miscarriage, gestational diabetes, hypertensive disease during pregnancy, preterm birth, cesarean section, and mood disorders. Lifestyle changes can improve the metabolic and endocrine consequences thus possibly improving infertility caused by anovulation.[1,2] Reaching a healthy weight before becoming pregnant will also improve the pregnancy outcome.

8.1. Are women with PCOS at increased risk of adverse pregnancy outcomes and why?

Draft recommendations:

8.1.1. Women with PCOS have an increased risk of adverse pregnancy outcomes, which should be identified during antenatal care. *(Moderate quality of evidence)*

8.1.2. Polycystic ovarian syndrome is associated with infertility, hyperandrogenemia, hyperinsulinemia with insulin resistance (IR), obesity, dyslipidemia, and chronic inflammation and these factors increase the risk of adverse pregnancy outcomes. *(High quality of evidence)*

8.1.3. Assisted reproductive technology in women with PCOS does not confer an additional risk of miscarriage, preterm birth, impaired fetal growth and cesarean section, over that observed in women without PCOS. *(Low quality of evidence)*

8.1.4. Polycystic ovarian syndrome women with pregnancy need increased surveillance during pregnancy and delivery to identify the risk factors of adverse pregnancy outcomes and prevent complications. *(Clinical practice point)*

Summary of evidence: Polycystic ovarian syndrome pregnancy has a higher risk of certain adverse pregnancy outcomes due to a combination of hormonal imbalances, metabolic issues, and other associated conditions and may not be directly related to the use of assisted reproductive technology (ART). Moreover, preconception with high BMI, hypertension, and impaired glucose tolerance may also influence pregnancy outcome. Infertility, hyperandrogenemia, hyperinsulinemia with insulin resistance (IR), obesity, dyslipidemia, and chronic inflammation can result in oxidative stress, epigenetic changes, defective trophoblastic invasion and placentation, disturbances in uterine blood flow, and also affect the oocyte and embryo quality which in turn result in pregnancy complications.[3] Placental dysfunction mediated by androgen excess and IR may lead to adverse pregnancy outcome and long-term developmental outcomes in offspring.

There is also a higher risk of preterm birth, admission to neonatal intensive care units (NICUs), and perinatal mortality and lower mean birthweight in offspring of women with PCOS, compared with offspring of women without PCOS, while fetal growth restriction, respiratory distress syndrome, and neonatal malformations appear similar.[2]

Research gap: The key research gaps include disparity in data regarding the impact of maternal characteristics such as age, BMI, and ART on pregnancy and neonatal outcomes. There is also substantial clinical heterogeneity in pooled analyses for multiple outcomes and insufficient studies that have performed subgroup analyses.[2] In many instances, PCOS is not identified during pregnancy which may then not recognize the risk factors for adverse birth outcomes.

8.2. What risks have been associated with pregnancy in women with PCOS and how do you prevent them?

Draft recommendations:

8.2.1. Pregnant women with PCOS have an increased risk of gestational weight gain, miscarriage, gestational diabetes, hypertensive disease during pregnancy, preeclampsia, intrauterine growth restriction, small for gestational age babies and low birth weight, preterm delivery, and cesarean section. *(Moderate quality of evidence)*

8.2.2. Early lifestyle intervention should be offered to pregnant women with PCOS, given the risk of higher baseline weight, impaired glucose tolerance, dyslipidemia, excess gestational weight gain, and pregnancy complications. *(Moderate quality of evidence)*

8.2.3. Preconceptional counseling, care, and preparation for pregnancy will prevent complications. *(Clinical practice point)*

8.2.4. Blood pressure measurement and OGTT should be performed when planning for a pregnancy or seeking fertility treatment. *(Clinical practice point)*

8.2.5. If OGTT is not performed in the preconception period, it should be done at the first antenatal visit and repeated at 24–28 weeks' gestation. *(Clinical practice point)*

8.2.6. Proper antenatal screening is helpful to diagnose and manage the adverse effects of pregnancy as early as possible. *(Clinical practice point)*

Summary of evidence: Obesity, placental thrombosis, endometrial defects, hyperandrogenemia, and insulin resistance are risk factors for pregnancy loss in PCOS women.[3] Higher AMH-levels seen in PCOS population with miscarriages. The chance of miscarriage increased by 90.8% for every 1 ng/mL increase in AMH level when AMH levels were more than 6.1 ng/mL.[3] PCOS morphology was not predictive of miscarriage or live birth.[4] Preterm birth and low birthweight remained higher in the offspring of women with PCOS and were associated with maternal PCOS, higher BMI, higher gestational weight gain, advanced maternal age, and ART pregnancies.[2] Insulin resistance and obesity which increase in TNF, IL-6, and leptin decrease in MCP-1 and is responsible for increased risk of gestational diabetes.[6]

A prediction model with five parameters (Type 2 diabetes mellitus in first-degree relatives, fasting glucose, fasting insulin, androstenedione, and SHBG) can accurately identify women with PCOS at risk for GDM before conception.[7] Odds of gestational hypertension were two to three times higher in women with PCOS compared with women without PCOS (OR: 2.20; 95% CI: 1.81, 2.69) and this was independent of ART.[2,8] Odds of preeclampsia were also higher in women with PCOS compared with women without PCOS (OR: 2.30; 95% CI: 1.87, 2.82).[2] The mechanisms involved in hypertensive disorders in pregnancy are increased oxidative stress, maternal vascular dysfunction, diffuse endothelial dysfunction due to IR, HA, atherosclerosis, alterations in inflammatory mediators abnormalities in the renin-angiotensin system and reduced placental perfusion.[9] There was no increase in instrumental deliveries though the odds for cesarean deliveries was significantly higher.[2]

There was a higher risk of GDM in phenotypes A, B, and C and a higher risk of PIH in phenotypes A and B and therefore women with these phenotypes need more precise prenatal care.[10] Higher incidence of PIH/HDP are directly related to androgen excess which results in endothelial dysfunction and atherosclerosis. [10]

Research gap: Most of the meta-analyses lacked power in sensitivity analyses due to the small number of studies per analysis and/or moderate-to-substantial heterogeneity. Moreover, meta-analyses of study-level aggregate data did not allow the evaluation of confounding effects or independent associations. However, these individual confounders could impact the results.[5] Moreover, significantly poor recognition of PCOS during pregnancy did not allow appropriate monitoring and support throughout the pregnancy. Addressing these gaps will help in a better understanding of the etiology for prevention, screening, and managing the complications. Pregnancy and PCOS-related research help to take steps to prevent pregnancy-related adverse effects. But still, several gaps remain in understanding the risks. More studies are needed on the subtypes and genetics of PCOS to determine the group who are at an increased risk of complications.

8.3. Should Insulin sensitizers be given prophylactically to prevent complications of pregnancy?

Draft recommendations:

8.3.1. Healthcare professionals should be aware that metformin in pregnant women with PCOS has not been shown to prevent:
- Gestational diabetes
- Late miscarriage (12 weeks +1 day to 21 weeks +6 days gestational age)
- Hypertension in pregnancy
- Preeclampsia
- Macrosomia or birthweight ≥4,000 g

8.3.2. Metformin could be considered in some circumstances (e.g., risk for preterm birth), to reduce preterm delivery and limit excess gestational weight gain, in pregnant women with PCOS. *(Moderate quality of evidence)*

8.3.3. Women should be counseled that the consequences of metformin exposure on long-term offspring health remain unclear and there is a suggestion of increased childhood weight, although causality is not certain. *(Clinical practice point)*

8.3.4. Clinicians should know about transplacental and endometrial transmission of insulin sensitizers and when to start and when to stop during pregnancy. *(Low quality of evidence)*

8.3.5. Clinicians should discuss with the patients about the side effects of insulin sensitizers. *(Clinical Practice point)*

Summary of evidence: Due to the increasing incidence of maternal obesity, GDM and type 2 diabetes, metformin use in pregnancy is increasing as its safety and efficacy has been demonstrated by several RCTs. The use of metformin has many maternal advantages when taken during and after pregnancy, including reduced maternal gestational weight gain, PTD and insulin requirements, a reduction in operative delivery and possible reduction in hypertensive disorders and future type 2 diabetes.[11] Some of these benefits may be even greater for women with a BMI ≥30 kg/m^2.[11] Several RCTs have demonstrated similar pregnancy outcomes as insulin therapy with less maternal weight gain and a high degree of patient compliance both in women with type 2 diabetes mellitus as well as those who are PCOS and nondiabetic and obese.[12] Metformin can be safely added to insulin in those women whose sugars are inadequately controlled with insulin alone. When used in combination with insulin it allows lower doses of insulin to be used.[12] There was no increase in the incidence of congenital malformations or miscarriages even when metformin is started before pregnancy and continued to term.[12]

In the international guidelines on PCOS published in 2023, metformin did not demonstrate improvement in any parameters except for preterm births.[1] The infant can also benefit from metformin use as it is associated with reduced rates of miscarriage, fetal growth retardation, macrosomia, hypoglycemia, and need for intensive neonatal unit care.

Research gap: Several knowledge gaps are identified in use of insulin sensitizers prophylactically in women with PCOS to prevent pregnancy complications. The studies focusing on gestational diabetes (GDM), glucose homeostasis, preeclampsia, hypertension, miscarriage, and gestational weight gain in women with PCOS had a high risk of bias, were underpowered and many were not blinded and therefore should be interpreted with caution. These methodological issues may impact the reliability of the results. The reduction in preeclampsia seen in the MOP trial is intriguing and needs further study.

Addressing these research gaps would help to give a proper recommendation on the use of metformin during pregnancy in women with PCOS. Until there are evidence-based answers to several uncertainties surrounding metformin use, women should be well informed about the risks and benefits and personalized, patient-centred approach should be employed to ensure the best outcome for both mother and child.

8.4. How obesity adds to the complications in pregnancy?

Draft recommendations:

8.4.1. Obesity in PCOS is primarily associated with increased risk of HDP, GDM, and operative deliveries when compared to women with PCOS and BMI <30 kg/m^2. *(Low quality of evidence)*

8.4.2. Diet and lifestyle modifications to optimize weight-control before pregnancy and adjusting treatment for comorbidities is of importance. *(Clinical practice point)*

Summary of evidence: Obesity and central adiposity are significantly higher in women with PCOS as compared to those without PCOS. Moreover, weight strongly influences the clinical severity of PCOS. PCOS combined with insulin resistance of obesity augments the risks of pregnancy complications which are associated with defects in insulin-mediated glucose uptake.

Once pregnant, obese PCOS women have significantly increased risk of pregnancy-related complications including gestational diabetes, hypertensive disorders, premature delivery, instrumental delivery and delivery by cesarean section.[13] Prepregnancy overweight/obesity in women with PCOS is associated with early fetal loss.[14] Obesity increases the chronic inflammatory mediators which adversely cause pregnancy-induced hypertension which in turn is related to maternal and fetal adverse outcomes.[13]

Research gap: High BMI is an independent risk factor for most pregnancy complications and inferior pregnancy outcome. But, in PCOS women, it is still debated whether PCOS per se or obesity has a negative impact on pregnancy with increased complication rate. Longitudinal studies on age and BMI-matched women with PCOS and controls are necessary to know the exact impact of obesity on pregnancy in PCOS women.

CONCLUSION

Polycystic ovarian syndrome women have a higher risk for adverse pregnancy outcomes and therefore the clinician should ensure proper identification of PCOS status early in pregnancy for appropriate monitoring and support throughout the pregnancy. Pregnancy in women with PCOS has metabolic, hormonal, and reproductive challenges. A comprehensive management is essential with early screening, proper and regular antenatal check-ups, and specific interventions when necessary to assess the maternal and fetal conditions. Multidisciplinary approaches may be essential to manage these patients.

KEYPOINTS

- Polycystic ovarian syndrome women are more likely to experience pregnancy complications, which are independent of but likely to be exacerbated by increased age and BMI and by assisted conception.
- Higher odds of miscarriage, GDM, gestational hypertension, preeclampsia, preterm delivery, and cesarean section are probably independent of age and BMI.
- Induced and/or operative deliveries are indicated in high-risk pregnancies for mothers or offspring.
- Babies born from women with PCOS may have increased morbidity and mortality.
- Underlying conditions and the interventions may both increase the risk of hemorrhage, infection, and rehospitalization.
- One must consider PCOS as a risk factor for pregnancy complications in preconception and in antenatal care guidelines to enable timely screening, proper monitoring, and early intervention.

REFERENCES

1. Teede HJ, Tay CT, Laven JJ, et al. Recommendations from the 2023 international evidence-based guideline for the assessment and management of polycystic ovary syndrome. Eur J Endocrinol. 2023;189(2):G43-64.
2. Bahri Khomami M, Shorakae S, Hashemi S, et al. Systematic review and meta-analysis of pregnancy outcomes in women with polycystic ovary syndrome. Nature communications. 2024;15(1):5591.
3. Wartena R, Matjila M. Polycystic ovary syndrome and recurrent pregnancy loss, a review of literature. Front Endocrinol. 2023;14:1183060.
4. Sha T, Wang X, Cheng W, et al. A meta-analysis of pregnancy-related outcomes and complications in women with polycystic ovary syndrome undergoing IVF. Reprod Biomed Online. 2019;39(2):281-93.
5. Khomami MB, Teede HJ. Addressing polycystic ovary syndrome in pregnancy care to improve outcomes. JAMA Network Open. 2024;7(8):e2430549.
6. Blumer I, Hadar E, Hadden DR, et al. Diabetes and pregnancy: an endocrine society clinical practice guideline. J Clin Endocrinol Metabol. 2013;98(11):4227-49.
7. de Wilde MA, Lamain-de Ruiter M, Veltman-Verhulst SM, et al. Increased rates of complications in singleton pregnancies of women previously diagnosed with polycystic ovary syndrome predominantly in the hyperandrogenic phenotype. Fertil Steril. 2017;108(2):333-40.
8. De Wilde MA, Veltman-Verhulst SM, Goverde AJ, et al. Preconception predictors of gestational diabetes: a multicentre prospective cohort study on the predominant complication of pregnancy in polycystic ovary syndrome. Hum Reprod. 2014;29(6):1327-36.
9. Chatzakis C, Tsakmaki E, Psomiadou A, et al. Different pregnancy outcomes according to the polycystic ovary syndrome diagnostic criteria: a systematic review and meta-analysis of 79 studies. Fertil Steril. 2022;117(4):854-81.
10. Firoozabadi AD, Firouzabadi RD, Eftekhar M, et al. Maternal and neonatal outcomes among pregnant women with different polycystic ovary syndrome phenotypes: a cross-sectional study. Int J Reprod Biomed. 2020;18(5):339.
11. Newman C, Dunne FP. Metformin for pregnancy and beyond: the pros and cons. Diab Med. 2022;39(3):e14700.
12. Hyer S, Balani J, Shehata H. Metformin in pregnancy: mechanisms and clinical applications. Int J Molecul Sci. 2018;19(7):1954.
13. Joham AE, Palomba S, Hart R. Polycystic ovary syndrome, obesity, and pregnancy. Semin Reprod Med. 2016;34(2):093-101.
14. Yang ST, Liu CH, Ma SH, et al. Association between pre-pregnancy overweightness/obesity and pregnancy outcomes in women with polycystic ovary syndrome: a systematic review and meta-analysis. Int J Environ Res Pub Health. 2022;19(15):9094.

CHAPTER 9

Long-term Health Implications and Comorbidities of PCOS

Sudhaa Sharma, Asna Beg Ashraf

INTRODUCTION

Polycystic ovary syndrome (PCOS) is a complex metabolic-endocrine disorder affecting women at various stages of life, with a global prevalence of approximately 10%–13%.[1] Women with PCOS face a significantly higher risk of developing a range of long-term health conditions and co-morbidities compared to those without the syndrome. These include cardiovascular, metabolic, endocrine, and psychological disorders, with many conditions occurring earlier and more frequently in women with PCOS.

Dyslipidemia, insulin resistance (IR), obesity, impaired glucose tolerance (IGT), hypertension (HTN), and metabolic syndrome (MetS) are highly prevalent in women with PCOS, exposing them to a higher risk of long-term metabolic sequelae like type 2 diabetes (T2D) and cardiovascular disease (CVD).[2]

9.1. What is the prevalence of long-term health implications and comorbidities?

Draft recommendations:

9.1.1. Clinicians should be aware that women with PCOS have an increased risk of HTN, T2D, cardiovascular disease, nonfatal cerebrovascular disease events, and adverse lipid profiles compared to those without PCOS. *(High quality of evidence)*

9.1.2. Women diagnosed with PCOS should be counseled about the possible *long-term health implications and comorbidities. (Clinical practice point)*

9.1.3. Clinicians should screen women with PCOS at diagnosis for impaired glucose tolerance, hypertension and hyperlipidemia and schedule regular follow-ups based on initial results and risk factors. *(Clinical practice point)*

Summary of evidence:

- A meta-analysis found that the prevalence of HTN in women with PCOS was 13.3% versus 6.6% in controls. The prevalence of T2D was 5.9% in women with PCOS compared to 2.0% in controls. Nonfatal cerebrovascular disease events and adverse lipid profile were also higher, but no significant differences were found for coronary disease events.[3]

- Nonobese women with PCOS also suffer from metabolic disturbances like hyperinsulinemia, IR, IGT, hypertriglyceridemia, and low HDL-C and the risk of long-term metabolic complications as shown by a meta-analysis.[4]

Research gaps:

1. Determining the true risk of other comorbidities is challenging due to various influencing factors, and the lack of long-term studies.
2. It is not yet clear whether women with differences in PCOS phenotypes and ethnic backgrounds have the same risks for the long-term consequences.
3. There is a need for long-term Indian studies.

9.2. Impaired glucose tolerance and type 2 diabetes—prevention, diagnosis, and management?

Draft recommendations:

9.2.1. Clinicians should inform women with PCOS about their increased risk of impaired fasting glucose, IGT and T2D regardless of age and BMI. *(High quality of evidence)*

9.2.2. Glycemic status should be evaluated at diagnosis of PCOS and rechecked every 1–3 years, based on individual risk factors for T2D. *(Moderate quality of evidence)*

9.2.3. Clinicians should recommend the 75 g OGTT to all women with PCOS, regardless of BMI. If an OGTT cannot be performed, FPG or HbA1C may be done, although their accuracy would be significantly lower. FPG is more sensitive than HbA1C. *(Low quality of evidence)*

9.2.4. An OGTT should be advised to all women with PCOS and without preexisting diabetes when planning a pregnancy or seeking fertility treatment. If preconception OGTT is not performed, it should be performed at the first antenatal visit. All women with PCOS should be tested at 24–28 weeks of gestation. *(Low quality of evidence)*

9.2.5. The key intervention to prevent progression to T2D, especially in those who are overweight and obese, are lifestyle modifications comprising dietary interventions and physical activity. *(Clinical practice point)*

9.2.6. The use of insulin-sensitizing agents, along with lifestyle interventions may improve their metabolic profile. *(Clinical practice point)*

Summary of evidence:

- Impaired FPG, IGT, and T2D are more prevalent in women with PCOS regardless of BMI status.[3,4]
- In a recent meta-analysis Belsti Y et al., (2024) concluded that using an HbA1C cut-off of ≥6.5% may misdiagnose half of the women with T2D. The 75 g OGTT is the most accurate test to assess glycemic status in PCOS, regardless of BMI. If OGTT is not possible, FBG or HbA1C may be considered, although their accuracy would be significantly lower.[1,5]

- The key intervention for preventing the progression to T2D, especially for obese or overweight women is lifestyle modification, comprising diet and physical activity.[1,6]
- A meta-analysis showed the significant impact of diet on improving IR and body composition by reduction of fasting insulin, FPG, BMI, weight, and WC.[7]
- A meta-analysis concluded that high-intensity interval training (achieving >90% of the individual's maximum heart rate) three times a week for ≥10 weeks effectively reduces IR and BMI in women with PCOS.[6]
- Metformin is associated with significantly lower 2-hour post-glucose load levels and reduction in FPG compared to placebo, but it has a negligible effect on weight. In women intolerant to metformin, thiazolidinediones (TZDs) were more effective in reducing FPG levels than placebo. The glucagon-like peptide-1 (GLP-1) receptor agonists are an attractive option for obese women due to their antidiabetic and weight-lowering properties. Liraglutide with metformin was associated with significant improvements in basal and postload glucose levels. Myo-inositol was associated with lower levels of insulin, glucose, and IR compared to placebo, metformin, or estrogen treatments.[8]

Research gaps:

1. Not all women with PCOS are overweight or obese; the impact of diet independent of weight loss needs to be investigated further.
2. Long-term Indian studies are needed on this aspect because the prevalence of T2D in Indian women is very high.

9.3. How to prevent, diagnose and manage cardiovascular risks?

Draft recommendations:

9.3.1. Women with PCOS should be informed about increased CVD risk and the potential of cardiovascular mortality and should be screened for its risk factors. *(Moderate quality of evidence)*

9.3.2. At diagnosis, women with PCOS should have a lipid profile (cholesterol, LDL-C, HDL-C and triglyceride level). Test frequency should be determined by the presence or absence of hyperlipidemia and additional risk factors. *(Moderate quality of evidence)*

9.3.3. Women with PCOS should have BP and weight measured at least once a year. *(Low quality of evidence)*

9.3.4. Clinicians should inform women with PCOS that lifestyle interventions is the first-line approach in modifying the risk of CVD. Adherence to a healthy diet, regular exercise, and weight reduction are the key components of prevention. *(Clinical practice point)*

9.3.5. Metformin, glucagon-like peptide-1 receptor agonists and SGLT-2 inhibitors may reduce CVD risk in insulin-resistant women by improving lipid profile and BMI. *(Moderate quality of evidence)*

9.3.6. If HTN is diagnosed in women with PCOS it should be controlled to reduce the risk of CVD. The target blood pressure should be <130/80 mm Hg. *(Clinical practice point)*

Summary of evidence:

- A recent meta-analysis found that oligomenorrhea/menstrual irregularity was associated with an increased risk of CVD, CHD, and MI, but not cerebrovascular disease. These associations remained consistent after adjusting for obesity.[9]
- A meta-analysis by Ramezani Tehrani F et al., (2020) showed that PCOS patients had a higher prevalence for CVD events, in all age groups. However, in population-based studies, only reproductive-age PCOS patients had a significantly higher risk. No significant difference in CVD event risk between menopausal/ageing PCOS women and healthy controls was found.
- A meta-analysis by Wekker et al., (2020) concluded that reproductive and premenopausal years are periods of increased CVD risk potentially due to a higher prevalence of obesity and T2D.
- Despite a lack of RCTs on the effectiveness of CVD risk screening in women with PCOS, the latest international guideline recommends regular screening for all PCOS women, regardless of BMI and advises annual BP and weight checks for women with traditional CVD risk factors every 1–3 years.[1]
- A meta-analysis by Amiri M et al. (2020) confirmed an elevated risk of HTN in pre-menopausal women with PCOS. However, after menopause, a history of PCOS may not significantly predispose to developing HTN.
- In a meta-analysis of patients with T2D, SGLT-2 inhibitors were linked to weight loss, improved glycemic control, and better CVD outcomes, including fewer heart failures, hospitalizations and mortality.[10]

Research gaps:

1. Evidence is still not clear on whether women with PCOS have a higher risk of CVD independent of established CVD risk factors.
2. PCOS tends to improve with age and CVD risk in older women with PCOS does not appear to be very different from those without PCOS. Data is limited and further studies are needed.
3. It is not known whether the presence of metabolic syndrome in women with PCOS is a risk for CVD in older women.
4. Future Indian clinical trials are needed to evaluate whether cardiometabolic screening and management in women with PCOS can reduce future CVD morbidity.

9.4. What are the criteria to diagnose metabolic syndrome?

Draft recommendations:

9.4.1. Women with PCOS should be informed and screened for MetS and its complications, especially CVD and T2D. *(High quality of evidence)*

9.4.2. Clinicians should be aware that early diagnosis and treatment of MetS may have a significant impact in reducing mortality and morbidity. *(High quality of evidence)*

9.4.3. For diagnosing metabolic syndrome three out of five criteria of the following should be present (NCEP-ATP III criteria). *(High quality of evidence)*

- Elevated triglycerides: ≥150 mg/dL
- Reduced HDL-C: <50 mg/dL
- Elevated blood pressure: Systolic ≥130 mm Hg and/or
Diastolic ≥85 mm Hg
or treated hypertension
- Elevated fasting glucose: >100 mg/dL
- *Elevated waist circumference:*
  Central/South American, Chinese, Japanese, South Asian: ≥80 cm
  Mediterranean, Middle East, Sub-Saharan African: ≥80 cm
  Europid (includes Canada, Europe, and the United States): ≥88 cm

Summary of evidence:

- A meta-analysis found that the prevalence of MetS in women with PCOS is significantly high, hence the importance of screening and treatment to prevent CVD.[11]
- For diagnosing metabolic syndrome, a joint interim statement, was issued by the IDF AHA/NHLBI and others.[12] The presence of any three of the following five criteria is required to diagnose MetS:
  - Abdominal obesity (WC >80 cm in women for Asians)
  - Elevated triglyceride levels (≥150 mg/dL)
  - Reduced levels of HDL-C or treatment for this disorder (HDL < 50 mg/dL in women)
  - High blood pressure (≥130/85 mm Hg)
  - Abnormal fasting glucose or previously diagnosed T2D (≥100 mg/dL)

Research gaps:

1. It remains uncertain whether metabolic syndrome can be considered a stand-alone condition.
2. The associations of metabolic syndrome with other comorbidities like NAFLD, sleep disorders, etc., require further investigations and long-term Indian studies.

9.5. Does the incidence of gynecological malignancies (endometrium, ovaries, and breast) increase in PCOS?

Draft recommendations:

9.5.1. Clinicians should be aware that premenopausal women with PCOS have a higher risk of developing atypical hyperplasia and endometrial cancer. *(High quality of evidence)*

9.5.2. Inform women with PCOS of their higher risk for atypical hyperplasia and endometrial cancer. However, since the overall risk of developing endometrial cancer is low, routine screening is not advised *(Clinical practice point)*

9.5.3. Long-standing untreated amenorrhea, obesity, type 2 diabetes and persistent thickened endometrium are risk factors for endometrial hyperplasia and endometrial cancer in women with PCOS. *(Clinical practice point)*

9.5.4. Clinicians should be aware that the association of PCOS with ovarian cancer is undetermined. *(Clinical practice point)*

9.5.5. Clinicians should be aware that the association of PCOS with breast cancer is low. *(Moderate quality of evidence)*

9.5.6. Clinicians should be aware that the association of PCOS with cervical, fallopian tube and vulvar cancer is undetermined. *(Clinical practice point)*

Summary of evidence:

- Li Z et al. (2022) in their meta-analysis found that PCOS was significantly associated with endometrial cancer (EC), but not with ovarian or breast cancer. However, in subgroups of high-quality studies, cohort studies, younger women (<54 years or premenopausal), and studies with unadjusted BMI, PCOS patients had a significantly higher risk of ovarian cancer.[13]
- A meta-analysis demonstrated four times greater odds of developing EC in women with PCOS, compared to controls. When postmenopausal women were excluded, the odds increased further.[14]
- A meta-analysis by Shobeiri F et al. (2019) found that PCOS does not increase the risk of breast cancer. Regarding the association of PCOS with cervical, fallopian tube and vulvar cancer the quality of evidence is heterogeneous.[15]

Research gaps:

1. The evidence linking PCOS to EC is weakened by inconsistent PCOS diagnosis, selection bias, and confounding factors like high BMI. More large-scale Indian prospective studies are needed to clarify this association and account for these variables.
2. The research linking PCOS to cancers of the cervix, fallopian tubes, and vulva is inconsistent.

9.6. How to prevent cancer risk in women with PCOS?

Draft recommendations:

9.6.1. Women with PCOS should be informed about preventive measures, including weight management, menstrual cycle regulation, and regular progesterone therapy to induce withdrawal bleeding at least every 3 months. *(Clinical practice point)*

9.6.2. When excessive endometrial thickness is detected, a biopsy with histological analysis and a withdrawal bleed should be considered. *(Clinical practice point)*

9.6.3. Progesterone should always be part of menopausal hormone therapy (MHT) in women with an intact uterus for endometrial protection, except in low dose vaginal estrogen therapy. *(Clinical practice point)*

Summary of evidence:

- Obesity is the most significant modifiable risk factor for EC. The aim should be to attain and maintain a healthy BMI (<25 kg/m^2). Exercise for 30 min a day, 5 days a week (moderate/vigorous intensity) is recommended. Breastfeeding should be encouraged. Coffee intake should be limited, and smoking avoided.[16]
- In the Nurses' Health Study II, OCs were linked to a lower risk of EC, regardless of the time since their last use.[17]
- The use of OCs confers long-term protection against EC. A meta-analysis found that, 10 years of use of OCs was estimated to reduce the absolute risk of EC arising before age 75 from 2·3 to 1·3 per 100 women.[18]
- Inducing regular withdrawal bleeding with cyclical hormones effectively reduces EC risk in women with PCOS. The LNG-IUS and high-dose oral progestogens are fertility-sparing treatment options for EC prevention in women with atypical hyperplasia (AH).[16]
- A scoping review found ample evidence demonstrating a risk reduction in women with obesity undergoing bariatric surgery for subsequent development of EC.[19]

Research gaps: Future research should focus on identifying patient groups at particularly high risk of developing EC and determining whether risk-reducing interventions could have a significant impact on prevention.

9.7. How do you manage endometrial cancer conservatively?

Draft recommendations:

9.7.1. Women with PCOS suffering from atypical hyperplasia or grade 1 endometrioid endometrial cancer without myometrial invasion should be counseled that fertility-sparing treatment is not the standard of care. Only those who strongly desire to preserve fertility should pursue this option. *(Low quality of evidence)*

9.7.2. Patients who are candidates for fertility-preserving treatment must be referred to specialized centers or experienced gyne-oncologists using well-defined protocols. *(Clinical practice point)*

Summary of evidence:

- Since many patients with PCOS are young or nulliparous at diagnosis, fertility-sparing therapy can be an option for highly selected patients with low-risk disease.[20]
- The selection criteria of patients according to the different world guidelines are as follows:[20,21] (All five criteria must be met.)
    i. Patients with AH or grade 1 endometrioid EC on endometrial biopsy—preferably through hysteroscopy, confirmed by an expert pathologist.
    ii. Tumor confined to the endometrium by imaging—pelvic MRI (preferred), expert TVS can be a substitute.
    iii. Absence of suspicious or metastatic disease on imaging.
    iv. No contraindications to HT, pregnancy, or genetic risk factors.
    v. Patients are to be counseled that fertility-sparing treatment is not the standard of care. Only those who strongly desire to preserve fertility should pursue this option.
- Hysteroscopic resection can potentially improve the success rate of fertility-preserving treatment of EC and AH.[22]
- Continuous progestin-based therapy which is the mainstay of conservative management may include megestrol acetate, medroxyprogesterone, or an intrauterine device containing levonorgestrel (LNG-IUS).[20]
- In a meta-analysis women <45 years with BMI <30 kg/m^2 achieved a high complete response rate of 84.6% with follow-ups of at least 24 months after LNG-IUS based therapies of endometrioid EC.[23]
- Combination of LNG-IUS with oral progestins with/without GnRH analogs can also be considered. Metformin appears to improve overall survival and reduce relapse risk in EC patients.[21]
- Follow-up is by biopsy and imaging at 3 and 6 months to assess response. After a complete response, conception is encouraged. Follow-up is recommended every 6 months (TVS and physical examination). Biopsy is recommended only in case of AUB/abnormal TVS. TH/BSO with staging is recommended: (i) after childbearing, (ii) if no response after 6 months on progestin therapy, or (iii) documented progression on biopsy.[20,21]

Research gaps:

1. Differences in demographic characteristics, such as older age and higher BMI, likely contribute to varying clinical outcomes, which may be associated with worse oncological outcomes.
2. Future Indian clinical studies should consider these individual differences in conservatively managing EC patients.

9.8. Is there an increased risk of inflammation in PCOS?

Draft recommendations:

9.8.1. Clinicians should be aware that low-grade chronic inflammation overlaps with comorbidities like CVD, dyslipidemia, obesity, and reproductive abnormalities in women with PCOS. *(Moderate quality of evidence)*

9.8.2. Clinicians should be aware that various inflammatory markers are implicated in the pathophysiology, and considered as biomarkers of PCOS. *(Low quality of evidence)*

Summary of evidence:

- The relationship between PCOS and inflammation is complex. A meta-analysis concluded that circulating CRP levels are moderately elevated in women with PCOS, independent of obesity, and indicating low-grade chronic inflammation.[24]
- Chronic inflammation overlaps with comorbidities such as CVD, dyslipidemia, obesity, and reproductive abnormalities in women with PCOS. Systemic and local chronic low-grade inflammation can increase oxidative stress in the ovary, negatively impacting folliculogenesis in PCOS.[25]
- Increased levels of various inflammatory markers have been observed in women with PCOS compared to age- and BMI-matched controls.[26]

Research gaps: Further studies are needed to establish the role of chronic inflammation in various aspects of PCOS pathophysiology and develop simplified diagnostic test to identify inflammation.

9.9. What is the prevalence, diagnosis and management of NAFLD and NASH in women with PCOS?

Draft recommendations:

9.9.1. Clinicians should be highly vigilant and initiate, implement and adjust screening practices to reflect the incidence of NAFLD in PCOS women of all ages and BMI categories. *(Moderate quality of evidence)*

9.9.2. A gastroenterologist/hepatologist should be involved in the care of women diagnosed with elevated liver enzymes or hepatic steatosis on imaging. *(Clinical practice point)*

Summary of evidence:

- A meta-analysis by Falzarano C et al., (2021) presented the worldwide prevalence of NAFLD in women with PCOS (51.56%) compared with women without PCOS (29.64%) ($p < 0.001$).
- Metabolic dysfunction-associated steatotic liver disease (MASLD) is the new term proposed (2023) to replace NAFLD. PCOS is linked to MASLD through IR, chronic inflammation, genetic factors, hyperandrogenemia, obesity, and gut microbiota imbalances.[27]

- Ultrasound is recommended as the first-line screening tool for detecting steatosis. Other chronic liver diseases or causes of steatosis have to be ruled out. Advanced fibrosis can be effectively identified using the NAFLD-fibrosis score, or by transient elastography.[28]
- For patients with PCOS and MASLD, regular monitoring of weight, glucose, and lipid metabolism is crucial. Lifestyle modifications are the recommended initial step. There are currently no approved drugs specifically for MASLD. Metabolism-related drugs, such as metformin, GLP-1 receptor agonists, and DPP-4 inhibitors, should be used based on each patient's circumstances and symptoms.[29]

Research gaps:

1. Further research is needed to understand the role of metabolism and how MASLD develops in women with PCOS. Combining molecular, epidemiological, and clinical data could lead to new ways to diagnose and treat MASLD in PCOS women.
2. Further studies are needed to prove that changes in gut microbiota directly cause MASLD and to develop precision treatments for MASLD targeting gut microbiota.
3. The incidence of MASLD in young and adolescent women has been largely overlooked. Research in this area lacks diversity, with most studies focusing on white women or lacking demographic details.

9.10. How will you prevent the occurrence of late sequelae in PCOS?

Draft recommendations:

9.10.1. Clinicians should recommend lifestyle changes, including diet, exercise, and weight loss, along with regular monitoring of glucose and lipid metabolism as the first line of treatment for women with PCOS to improve long-term outcomes. These changes should precede and/or accompany any pharmacological treatment. *(Low quality of evidence)*

9.10.2. Overweight or obese women should be counseled about the benefits of weight loss which include significantly reduced risk of CVD, T2D, MetS, OSA, EC, and NAFLD. In women with excess weight, a weight loss of 5–10% is advised, aiming for an energy deficit of 30% or 500–750 kcal/day (1,200–1,500 kcal/day). *(Clinical practice point)*

9.10.3. Clinicians should be aware that NAFLD is often reversible in its early stages, so early detection is crucial to prevent further liver damage and significantly improve the quality of life. *(Clinical practice point)*

9.10.4. Bariatric surgery may be considered for morbidly obese women with PCOS, particularly those with a BMI of 40 kg/m^2 or more, or 35 kg/m^2 or more with a high-risk obesity-related condition if standard weight loss strategies have not been successful. *(Moderate quality of evidence)*

Summary of evidence:

- In their meta-analysis, Wekker et al. (2020) suggest that early signs of PCOS, such as irregular menstrual cycles and infertility, provide a window of opportunity for preventing long-term cardiometabolic complications by increasing awareness of healthy lifestyle choices and offering support to improve modifiable factors like smoking and obesity.[30]
- A Cochrane review of 15 RCTs found that lifestyle interventions, compared to minimal intervention or usual care, significantly reduced weight and BMI.
- A meta-analysis found that bariatric surgery led to improvements in BMI, circulating glucose levels, IR, hyperandrogenism, HTN, related clinical symptoms, menstrual cycles, and ovulation rates.[31]
- Combining lifestyle management with pharmacotherapy can significantly improve metabolic profiles and reduce CVD risk. Statin therapy is recommended for women with PCOS and elevated atherosclerotic CVD risk. When CVD risk is unclear, measuring subclinical atherosclerosis, such as carotid plaque or coronary artery calcium, can aid in deciding on statin therapy. Medications like metformin and glucagon-like peptide-1 receptor agonists also effectively reduce CVD risk in insulin-resistant individuals.[2]

Research gaps:

1. Individualized and precise treatment of PCOS is challenging due to the lack of a clear understanding of etiology and prognostic markers.
2. The current guidelines focus on experimental symptom management and lack treatments based on underlying mechanisms.

CONCLUSION

Long-term health consequences and comorbidities associated with PCOS pose a significant challenge and an immense healthcare burden. Since gynecologists diagnose PCOS, they must have a comprehensive understanding of its long-term implications. It is crucial for providing holistic care that addresses not only the immediate symptoms but also the broader, long-term health challenges posed by PCOS. Counseling on long-term health consequences and co-morbidities is essential in PCOS management and should be a priority. Effective patient counseling leads to better clinical outcomes and patient satisfaction. Further research on long-term monitoring strategies and effective treatment for women with comorbid conditions associated with PCOS is needed. We also need large population-based studies on long-term consequences for Indian women.

ABBREVIATIONS

AC: Abdominal circumference
AH: Atypical hyperplasia
AHA: American Heart Association
BMI: Body mass index
BP: Blood pressure
CHD: Coronary heart disease
CPAP: Continuous positive airway pressure
CRP: C-reactive protein
CVD: Cardiovascular disease
DPP-4: Dipeptidyl peptidase IV
EC: Endometrial cancer
FPG: Fasting plasma glucose
GLP-1: Glucagon-like peptide-1
GnRH: Gonadotropin-releasing hormone
HbA1C: Hemoglobin A1C
HDL-C: High density lipoprotein-cholesterol
HT: Hormone therapy
HTN: Hypertension
IDF: International Diabetes Federation
IGT: Impaired glucose tolerance
IR: Insulin resistance
LDL-C: Low-density lipoprotein-cholesterol
LNG-IUS: Levonorgestrel-intrauterine system
MASLD: Metabolic dysfunction-associated steatotic liver disease
MetS: Metabolic syndrome
MHT: Menopause hormone therapy
MI: Myocardial infarction
NAFLD: Nonalcoholic fatty liver disease
NHLBI: National Heart, Lung and Blood Institute
OC: Oral contraceptive
OGTT: Oral glucose tolerance test
OSA: Obstructive sleep apnea
PCOS: Polycystic ovarian syndrome
PICO: Population, intervention, comparison, and outcomes
RCT: Randomized controlled trial
SGLT-2: Sodium-glucose transport protein 2
T2D: Type 2 diabetes
TG: Triglycerides
TH/BSO: Total hysterectomy/bilateral salpingo-oophorectomy
TSH: Thyroid stimulating hormone
TVS: Transvaginal scan
WC: Waist circumference

REFERENCES

1. Teede HJ, Tay CT, Laven JJE, et al. Recommendations from the 2023 international evidence-based guideline for the assessment and management of polycystic ovary syndrome. J Clin Endocrinol Metab. 2023;108(10):2447-69.
2. Guan C, Zahid S, Minhas AS, et al. Polycystic ovary syndrome: a "risk-enhancing" factor for cardiovascular disease. Fertil Steril. 2022;117(5):924-35.
3. Wekker V, van Dammen L, Koning A, et al. Long-term cardiometabolic disease risk in women with PCOS: a systematic review and meta-analysis. Hum Reprod Update. 2020;26(6):942-60.
4. Zhu S, Zhang B, Jiang X, et al. Metabolic disturbances in non-obese women with polycystic ovary syndrome: a systematic review and meta-analysis. Fertil Steril. 2019;111(1):168-77.
5. Belsti Y, Enticott J, Azumah R, et al. Diagnostic accuracy of oral glucose tolerance tests, fasting plasma glucose and haemoglobin A1c for type 2 diabetes in women with polycystic ovary syndrome: a systematic review and meta-analysis. Diabetes Metab Syndr. 2024;18(3):102970.
6. Santos IKD, Nunes FASS, Queiros VS, et al. Effect of high-intensity interval training on metabolic parameters in women with polycystic ovary syndrome: a systematic review and meta-analysis of randomized controlled trials. PLoS One. 2021;16:e0245023.
7. Shang Y, Zhou H, Hu M, et al. Effect of diet on insulin resistance in polycystic ovary syndrome. J Clin Endocrinol Metab. 2020;105(10):dgaa425.
8. Pani A, Gironi I, Di Vieste G, et al. From prediabetes to Type 2 diabetes mellitus in women with polycystic ovary syndrome: lifestyle and pharmacological management. Int J Endocrinol. 2020;2020:6276187.
9. Lo ACQ, Lo CCW, Oliver-Williams C. Cardiovascular disease risk in women with hyperandrogenism, oligomenorrhea/menstrual irregularity or polycystic ovaries (components of polycystic ovary syndrome): a systematic review and meta-analysis. Eur Heart J Open. 2023;3(4):oead 061.
10. McGuire DK, Shih WJ, Cosentino F, et al. Association of SGLT2 Inhibitors With Cardiovascular and Kidney Outcomes in Patients With Type 2 Diabetes: A Meta-analysis. JAMA Cardiol. 2021;6(2):148-58.
11. Otaghi M, Milad Azami, Ali Khorshidi, et al. The association between metabolic syndrome and polycystic ovary syndrome: a systematic review and meta-analysis. Diabetes Metab Syndr. 2019;13(2):1481-9.
12. Alberti KG, Eckel RH, Grundy SM, et al. International Diabetes Federation Task Force on Epidemiology and Prevention. National Heart, Lung, and Blood Institute. American Heart Association. World Heart Federation. International Atherosclerosis Society. International Association for the Study of Obesity. Harmonizing the metabolic syndrome: a joint interim statement of the International Diabetes Federation Task Force on Epidemiology and Prevention; National Heart, Lung, and Blood Institute; American Heart Association; World Heart Federation; International Atherosclerosis Society; and International Association for the Study of Obesity. Circulation. 2009;120(16):1640-5.
13. Li Z, Wang YH, Wang LL, et al. Polycystic ovary syndrome and the risk of endometrial, ovarian and breast cancer: an updated meta-analysis. Scott Med J. 2022;67(3):109-20.

14. Johnson JE, Daley D, Tarta C, et al. Risk of endometrial cancer in patients with polycystic ovarian syndrome: a meta analysis. Oncol Lett. 2023;25(4):168.
15. Shobeiri F, Jenabi E. The association between polycystic ovary syndrome and breast cancer: a meta-analysis. Obstet Gynecol Sci. 2016;59(5):367-72.
16. Njoku K, Abiola J, Russell J, et al. Endometrial cancer prevention in high-risk women. Best Pract Res Clin Obstet Gynaecol. 2020;65:66-78.
17. Burchardt NA, Shafrir AL, Kaaks R, et al. Oral contraceptive use by formulation and endometrial cancer risk among women born in 1947-1964: The Nurses' Health Study II, a prospective cohort study. Eur J Epidemiol. 2021;36(8):827-39.
18. Collaborative Group on Epidemiological Studies on Endometrial Cancer. Endometrial cancer and oral contraceptives: an individual participant meta-analysis of 27 276 women with endometrial cancer from 36 epidemiological studies. Lancet Oncol. 2015;16:1061-70
19. Aubrey C, Black K, Campbell S, et al. Endometrial cancer and bariatric surgery: a scoping review. Surg Obes Relat Dis. 2019;15(3):497-501.
20. Abu-Rustum N, Yashar C, Arend R, et al. Uterine Neoplasms, Version 1.2023, NCCN Clinical Practice Guidelines in Oncology. J Natl Compr Canc Netw. 2023;21(2):181-209.
21. Concin N, Matias-Guiu X, Vergote I, et al. ESGO/ESTRO/ESP guidelines for the management of patients with endometrial carcinoma. Radiother Oncol. 2021;154:327-53.
22. Bilir E, Kahramanoğlu İ. The role of hysteroscopy in fertility preservation in endometrial cancer and atypical endometrial hyperplasia: a semi-systematic literature review. Arch Gynecol Obstet. 2023;308(4):1113-26.
23. Wei H, Pan N, Zhang W, et al. Levonorgestrel-releasing intrauterine system-based therapies for early-stage endometrial cancer: a systematic review and meta-analysis. J Gynecol Oncol. 2023;34(2):e36.
24. Aboeldalyl S, James C, Seyam E, et al. The Role of Chronic inflammation in polycystic ovarian syndrome—a systematic review and meta-analysis. Int J Mol Sci. 2021;22:2734.
25. Velez LM, Seldin M, Motta AB. Inflammation and reproductive function in women with polycystic ovary syndrome. Biol Reprod. 2021;104(6):1205-17.
26. Rudnicka E, Suchta K, Grymowicz M, et al. Chronic low grade inflammation in pathogenesis of PCOS. Int J Mol Sci. 2021;22:3789.
27. Arvanitakis K, Chatzikalil E, Kalopitas G, et al. Metabolic dysfunction-associated steatotic liver disease and polycystic ovary syndrome: a complex interplay. J Clin Med. 2024;13:4243.
28. Papatheodoridi M, Cholongitas E. Diagnosis of Non-alcoholic Fatty Liver Disease (NAFLD): Current Concepts. Curr Pharm Des. 2018;24(38):4574-86.
29. Xu Q, Zhang J, Lu Y, et al. Association of metabolic-dysfunction associated steatotic liver disease with polycystic ovary syndrome. iScience. 2024;27(2):108783.
30. Wekker V, van Dammen L, Koning A, et al. Long-term cardiometabolic disease risk in women with PCOS: a systematic review and meta-analysis. Hum Reprod Update. 2020;26(6):942-60.
31. Li YJ, Han Y, He B. Effects of bariatric surgery on obese polycystic ovary syndrome: a systematic review and meta-analysis. Surg Obes Relat Dis. 2019;15(6):942-50.

CHAPTER 10

Patient's Education, Counseling, and Support Groups in Polycystic Ovary Syndrome

Anushree Devashish Patil, Deepti Tandon, Nupoor Rajendra Limaye

INTRODUCTION

Polycystic ovarian syndrome (PCOS) is a frequently occurring gynecological and metabolic disorder affecting women aged 15–49 years from adolescence through menopause and hence the condition requires a lifecycle approach.[1] PCOS has a changing women's health paradigm from an early age and extends into postmenopause. Apart from reproductive disorders, it is associated with long-term metabolic and cardiovascular disorders, thus requiring a multi-disciplinary approach. PCOS is primarily managed through lifestyle modifications and medication, with the help of proper education, information, and coping skills crucial for long-term management with inclusion of family members and also considering sociocultural factors. Previous research has shown that many individuals with PCOS experience a lack of sufficient information, have negative interactions with healthcare professionals, lengthy diagnostic processes, and a deficit in clinical, educational, and emotional support.[2] Recent research indicates that the prevalence of PCOS among women in India ranges from 8.2 to 22.5%.[3] Counseling is integral to PCOS management enabling enhanced clinical outcomes and patient satisfaction. Digital tools for education and PCOS support groups have built an opportunity for physicians to create awareness, help with timely diagnosis and overcome PCOS symptoms.

10.1. What are the characteristics of available models of care implemented in PCOS clinics or services?

Draft recommendations:

10.1.1. Healthcare systems should implement a multidisciplinary approach that includes specialists such as endocrinologists, gynecologists, dietitians, psychologists, dermatologists, and other relevant professionals to tackle PCOS's complex nature. *(Strong quality of evidence)*

10.1.2. Models should integrate psychological support and social interventions alongside medical treatments. *(Moderate quality of evidence)*

10.1.3. Adolescent-specific models of care (MoCs) that focus on education, lifestyle interventions, and individualized medical care should be initiated. *(Moderate quality of evidence)*

10.1.4. Care models should also be developed in the government healthcare system including primary health care which should include healthcare professional training, virtual options and appropriate referral linkages. *(Clinical practice point)*

Summary of evidence: A model of care (MoC) is a comprehensive framework for delivering care, created in collaboration with the end-users which adheres to evidence-based practices and established standards. A systematic review was undertaken by Melson et al. to identify models of care (MoCs) available for PCOS and to describe their characteristics and alignment with the International PCOS Guideline.[4] Out of 3,671 articles, six articles describing five MoCs which were included in this systematic review. All MoCs described a multidisciplinary approach, including an endocrinologist, dietitian, gynecologist, psychologist, dermatologist, and relevant professionals. Three MoCs described all aspects of PCOS care aligned with the International Guideline recommendations. These include providing education on long-term risks, lifestyle interventions, screening and management of emotional well-being, cardiometabolic diseases, and the dermatological and reproductive elements of PCOS. Three MoCs evaluated patient's outcomes, healthcare professionals' outcomes and satisfaction, with generally positive findings. This review cited the ICMR-NIRRCH MoC from India as one among the five MOCs that adhere to international evidence-based guidelines for PCOS.[5]

As per our review, we could identify the following types of MOCs for PCOS.

1. *Multidisciplinary MoC:* Several studies highlight the importance of a multidisciplinary MOC in PCOS management. It was demonstrated that incorporating long-term risk management, lifestyle modification, emotional support, cardiometabolic, dermatological, and reproductive care significantly benefits patients.[4,5] This approach ensures comprehensive care that addresses all aspects of the syndrome.
2. *Biopsychosocial model:* The biopsychosocial model focuses on the interplay between biological, social, and psychological factors.[6] This model aims to improve the overall quality of life (QoL) for PCOS patients by addressing not just the physical symptoms but also the emotional and social challenges they face.
3. *Specific models for adolescents:* Adolescents with PCOS have unique needs that require specialized care. An adolescent-specific model is implemented at the Children's Hospital Colorado. This model combines educational sessions with individual clinic visits, tailored to address the specific challenges faced by younger patients.[7]

Thus, the review of various models of care (MOC) implemented in PCOS clinics reveals a diverse approach to managing this condition, with a common theme of emphasizing multidisciplinary care. This includes the integration of various specialities such as gynecology, dermatology, psychology, and nutrition, which is essential in addressing the multifaceted nature of PCOS.

Research gap:

- There is limited literature describing PCOS MoCs in routine practice. Future research should explore developing costeffective cocreated multidisciplinary PCOS MoCs codesigned with women globally. This may be facilitated by the exchange of best practices between institutions with an established MoC and those who are interested in setting one up.
- There is a notable gap in the efficacy and long-term outcomes of these models, suggesting a need for further research to validate their effectiveness over time.
- Future efforts should focus on scaling up MoCs.

In conclusion, while various MoCs for PCOS clinics demonstrate promising results, ongoing evaluation and adaptation are essential to ensure these models meet the evolving needs of patients. The integration of multidisciplinary and biopsychosocial approaches appears to be the most effective in providing comprehensive care, yet continuous research and refinement are necessary to optimize these models for better patient's outcomes.

10.2. How can we best support women to navigate the impact of PCOS on family and

Draft recommendations:

10.2.1. Encourage family involvement in self-management as getting family members involved in PCOS self-management can dramatically improve women's support systems. *(Moderate quality of evidence)*

10.2.2. Implementing the biopsychosocial model which takes into account the biological, psychological, and social aspects of health has the potential to dramatically improve the QoL for women with PCOS. *(Moderate quality of evidence)*

10.2.3. To decrease the stigma and marginalization, public health educators need to boost societal awareness and education regarding PCOS. *(Clinical practice point)*

10.2.4. One needs to develop socioculturally sensitive resources and educational materials on PCOS for families of those affected by the condition. *(Clinical practice point)*

Summary of evidence: Polycystic ovary syndrome significantly affects a woman's life, including family and interpersonal relationships. Comprehensive support for women with PCOS should focus on self-management, family involvement, and behavioral changes. The biopsychosocial model, which considers biological, psychological, and social factors, is crucial for improving the well-being of women with PCOS by addressing its physical, emotional, and social impacts. Family involvement in self-management is essential, as it significantly aids in symptom management and promotes healthy lifestyle changes as emphasized by Young et al. (2020).[8]

Promoting healthy behaviors such as proper nutrition, regular exercise, stress management, and adherence to medical treatments is key to managing PCOS. Family involvement enhances these changes by providing a supportive environment. Support groups and counseling services offer platforms for women with PCOS and their families to share experiences, seek advice, and gain emotional support, reducing isolation and offering practical management strategies.[8]

Polycystic ovarian syndrome often leads women to alter their life plans, particularly regarding family planning. Women also manage other physical conditions and face significant mental health challenges, including depression and suicidal ideation. These findings underscore the complex impacts of PCOS and the need for comprehensive and compassionate support.[9]

Research gap:

- There is an inadequate research into the specific dynamics of family engagement, as well as how diverse family structures and cultural backgrounds influence the efficiency of support interventions.
- Present research ignores the possible long-term effects on both the individual with PCOS and their family members.
- More extensive research is needed on the challenges that women have in maintaining lifestyle changes, particularly in the context of their familial and social surroundings.

10.3. What are the key challenges for those with PCOS when interacting with healthcare professionals about PCOS and related features?

Draft recommendations:

10.3.1. Healthcare providers should be trained in shared decision-making to provide clear, comprehensive information about PCOS, including its symptoms, evidence-based treatment options, lifestyle modifications, counseling, emotional support, and a multidisciplinary approach. *(Strong quality of evidence)*

10.3.2. Healthcare providers should adhere to standard treatment guidelines and use appropriate resources by healthcare providers. *(Clinical practice point)*

10.3.3. Delays in diagnosis and treatment should be reduced by streamlining the diagnostic and referral process and enhancing early detection of PCOS in adolescents. *(Clinical practice point)*

10.3.4. Evidence-based strategies and resources can enhance patient's participation, which includes knowledge, skills, ability, confidence, and willingness to manage their own health and care. (Evidence-based International Guidelines for PCOS 2023). *(Clinical practice point)*

Summary of evidence: Polycystic ovary syndrome poses significant challenges in diagnosis and treatment, often leading to patient dissatisfaction. The diagnostic process is lengthy and complex, with many patients perceiving healthcare professionals as lacking knowledge, resulting in delayed diagnoses and worsening symptoms. This can increase anxiety, depression, and frustration among patients, negatively impacting their QoL.[2] Empathetic communication is often lacking, deepening dissatisfaction and exacerbating stigma, self-image issues, and mental health concerns. Adolescents face additional challenges due to the overlap of PCOS symptoms with normal puberty, further complicating diagnosis and treatment.[10] Many patients seek multiple healthcare options, including Allopathic, Homeopathic, and Ayurvedic care, but report dissatisfaction with the repetitive treatments and lack of guidance on lifestyle changes.[11] Enhanced healthcare professional knowledge and collaborative care efforts are essential for improving PCOS management.

Research gap:
- Requirement for culturally appropriate and tailored treatment programs.
- Current treatments frequently fail to address PCOS patients' holistic needs, which include hormonal, metabolic, and psychological factors. Patients typically report unhappiness with recurrent treatments and a lack of practical advice on lifestyle modifications, indicating a gap between physician recommendations and patient's execution.

10.4. How important are support groups and how do they function?

Draft recommendations:

10.4.1. Encourage PCOS support groups to provide evidence-based information, peer support, awareness and socioculturally relevant woman-centered care. *(Moderate quality of evidence)*

10.4.2. PCOS support should be encouraged to have long-standing partnerships with healthcare providers, professional agencies, and researchers, making substantial contributions to advocacy and raising awareness. *(Clinical practice point)*

Summary of evidence: Literature review of PubMed and Medline could retrieve very few articles on PCOS support groups. According to a study by Tolins et al. (2023), the Peer Outreach Support Team (POST) program, which trained 59 peer supporters across 11 departments in a two-hospital system, demonstrated the effectiveness of peer support.[12] Trained PCOS patients found the training useful and reported that their interactions with peers improved, with decreased negative emotions, and reduced stigma among their peers. Similarly, in PCOS support groups, peer support allows individuals to connect with others who have similar experiences, offering mutual encouragement and practical advice on managing the condition.[12]

Support groups can also enhance the knowledge and understanding of healthcare professionals regarding PCOS. It should be emphasized that there is a need for co-creating resources between healthcare professionals and individuals with PCOS to provide culturally appropriate and holistic care.[2] Support groups can serve as platforms for this co-creation, where healthcare providers and patients collaborate to improve care strategies and outcomes.

Effective lifestyle management for women with PCOS depends on being well-informed and supported.[13] Unfortunately, many women find their needs unmet by current healthcare services and available information.

Polycystic ovarian syndrome support groups offer evidence-based information, peer support, raise awareness, and advocate for woman-centered care. Women gain valuable information and emotional support from these groups, boosting their confidence in managing the condition. Some support groups partner with healthcare providers and researchers, significantly contributing to advocacy and awareness. There is a major opportunity for collaboration among healthcare providers, professional societies, and support groups to enhance the availability of evidence-based information through these groups.[13]

Numerous international English-speaking PCOS support groups are present online. Early research found that women seek both information and emotional support from these groups. A 2007 Australian study revealed that online support groups provide practical, accessible information, and validate women's experiences with PCOS. Participation in these groups reduces loneliness and offers helpful information, improving women's confidence in communicating with healthcare providers and managing their condition.

However, the study also noted potential drawbacks, such as distress from reading negative experiences and feelings of exclusion due to group dynamics. A moderator could potentially address these issues. Messages seeking socio-emotional support received emotional support, but requests for informational support were less frequently fulfilled.

Research on in-person support groups is less common but shows similar results. A study on a nurse-led UK support group found that women attended support groups for information and to connect with others with PCOS met their expectations and women reported feeling more empowered and better able to manage their condition.[13]

A study on social networking in online support groups for health shows that social media and patient support groups play a crucial role in providing emotional and informational support to patients. Patients selectively use different features of online support groups based on their motivations, with those seeking social interaction using a broader range of features like friending and blogging. In contrast, those focused on information tend to rely more on discussion boards. A study highlights the importance of tailoring online support group features to meet the diverse needs of users.[14]

Research gaps:

- Research studies to understand access and functioning to different types of support groups are lacking.
- Research studies on the outcome evaluation of support groups need to be undertaken.

10.5. Is a questionnaire necessary before counseling?

10.5.1. Out of the four databases—PubMed, Medline, Cochrane, and Scopus—we only utilized PubMed and Medline due to our access limitations. After conducting searches with the relevant keywords, we did not find any pertinent articles for this particular question.

10.6. Who should counsel women with PCOS?

Draft recommendations:

10.6.1. Implementing a multidisciplinary approach for PCOS counseling involves integrating various specialities and expertise to provide a comprehensive and holistic treatment plan. *(Moderate quality of evidence)*

10.6.2. Psychologists and trained counselors can counsel women with PCOS. *(Clinical practice point)*

Summary of evidence: Gynecologists and endocrinologists are essential in diagnosing and managing the medical aspects of PCOS, focusing on hormonal imbalances, reproductive health, and metabolic issues. According to Lathia et al., though medical treatment forms a significant component of managing PCOS, it must be integrated with other support services to address the multifaceted nature of the condition. The involvement of psychologists and psychiatrists is also crucial, as the psychosocial aspects of PCOS are often neglected. These professionals provide vital counseling to help patients to manage anxiety, depression, and body image issues commonly associated with PCOS, which is essential for holistic care and helps patients to cope with the emotional challenges of the condition.

Nutritionists and dietitians play a pivotal role in managing PCOS through dietary interventions. They offer personalized nutrition plans that help to regulate insulin levels, manage weight, and reduce the risk of comorbidities such as diabetes. Proper dietary guidance can also alleviate symptoms like hirsutism and acne, contributing to overall well-being.

Cosmetologists and dermatologists form an integral part of the team managing PCOS in addressing the physical symptoms of PCOS, such as hirsutism and acne, which can significantly impact a woman's self-esteem and body image. They provide treatments and skincare advice to manage these symptoms effectively. Counseling for women with PCOS should involve a multidisciplinary team to address the diverse aspects of the condition.

Research gap: Content of counseling for PCOS and effect of counseling on treatment outcome and adherence to treatment need to be researched.

10.7. Should the counseling be individual or in a group?

Draft of recommendations:

10.7.1. Individual counseling for personalized care is essential as it provides a tailored and personalized approach to care, which will ensure the unique needs and concerns of each person are addressed with specialized attention. *(Clinical practice point)*

10.7.2. Group counseling for community support and awareness is essential as it fosters a sense of community support and raises awareness, allowing participants to share experiences and insights in a collective environment that promotes mutual understanding and collective growth. *(Clinical practice point)*

Summary of evidence: Effective patient's education and counseling customized to women of all ages are critical. Improving psychological screening, diagnosis, and access to treatment can greatly enhance women's QoL with PCOS. There is an urgent need for research into effective treatment and long-term monitoring measures for women with co-morbidities in PCOS.

Lathia (2022) discusses the need for counseling at various stages of life.[6] Fertility advice is essential for women who are contemplating a pregnancy. For people who are not planning a pregnancy, counseling should concentrate on sexual health, self-esteem, self-image, assertiveness training, and problem-solving abilities. Person-centered guidance and family support are vital for women going through or coming out of menopause. The study suggests that counseling is essential for controlling PCOS across all age groups. Individual as well as group counseling plays a pivotal role in addressing different aspects of PCOS care.

Research gap:

- Despite the acknowledged importance of counseling in PCOS, significant research gaps exist. There has been little study into whether individual or group counseling is more useful for women with PCOS.
- Most studies emphasize the importance of counseling but do not compare the outcomes of various counseling forms.

- Furthermore, research frequently ignores the long-term impact of counseling on the psychological well-being of women with PCOS.
- There is also a scarcity of research into the exact aspects of counseling that contributes the most to improved outcomes.

10.8. Is patient's education an important aspect in managing PCOS?

Draft recommendations:

10.8.1. Implement comprehensive user-friendly patient's education programs including digital platforms which include multidisciplinary approach for the management of PCOS. *(Clinical practice point)*

10.8.2. Patient's education should include information regarding access to health care, comorbidities, follow-ups, and support groups. *(Clinical practice point)*

Summary of evidence: Polycystic ovarian syndrome management necessitates a multidisciplinary strategy that includes screening, assessment, and therapy. Counseling and patient's education are critical for treating the multiple challenges associated with PCOS.

Digital tools and support groups for PCOS have raised awareness, enabled quicker diagnosis, and aided with symptom management. However, specific guidelines on the psychosocial components of PCOS are still needed, emphasizing the necessity of patient's education and counseling in dealing with these different issues.[6]

Finally, patient's education is essential to PCOS management and should be recognized by all HCPs. Effective patient's counseling can result in improved therapeutic outcomes and increased satisfaction.

Research gaps:

- Availability and access to patient's education material which is socio-culturally relevant for different age groups.
- Effect of patient's education on adherence to treatment

CONCLUSION

Polycystic ovarian syndrome is a common and distressing condition in which women often lack adequate support and information to achieve the best health and well-being outcomes. Counseling is an integral part of PCOS management and optimum patient's counseling would enable overall enhanced clinical outcomes and patient's satisfaction.[15] Counseling and support groups improve QoL, assist with fertility, and reduce the risk of long-term health problems. Support groups provide relevant information, raise awareness, and provide social and emotional support. Counseling by doctors and support groups helps in improving the confidence and ability to manage their condition with distress.

REFERENCES

1. Gu Y, Zhou G, Zhou F, et al. Life Modifications and PCOS: Old Story But New Tales. Front Endocrinol. 2022;13:808898.
2. Lau GM, Elghobashy M, Thanki M, et al. A systematic review of lived experiences of people with polycystic ovary syndrome highlights the need for holistic care and co-creation of educational resources. Front Endocrinol. 2022;13:1064937.
3. Siddiqui S, Mateen S, Ahmad R, et al. A brief insight into the etiology, genetics, and immunology of polycystic ovarian syndrome (PCOS). J Assisted Reprod Genet. 2022;39(11):2439-73.
4. Melson E, Davitadze M, Malhotra K, et al. A systematic review of models of care for polycystic ovary syndrome highlights the gap in the literature, especially in developing countries. Front Endocrinol (Lausanne). 2023;14:1217468.
5. Patil AD, Vaidya RA, Begum S, et al. An integrated multidisciplinary model of care for addressing comorbidities beyond reproductive health among women with polycystic ovary syndrome in India. Indian J Med Res. 2022;156(3):449-58.
6. Lathia T, Joshi A, Behl A, et al. A Practitioner's toolkit for polycystic ovary syndrome counselling. Indian J Endocrinol Metabol. 2022;26(1):17-25.
7. Torres-Zegarra C, Sundararajan D, Benson J, et al. Care for adolescents with polycystic ovary syndrome: development and prescribing patterns of a multidisciplinary clinic. J Pediatr Adoles Gynecol. 2021;34(5):617-25.
8. Young CC, Sagna AO, Monge M, et al. Theoretically grounded exploration of individual and family self-management of polycystic ovary syndrome in adolescents. Compr Child Adolesc Nurs. 2020;43(4):348-62.
9. Williams S, Sheffield D, Knibb RC. The polycystic ovary syndrome quality of life scale (PCOSQOL): development and preliminary validation. Health Psychol Open. 2018;5(2):2055102918788195.
10. Meczekalski B, Niwczyk O, Kostrzak A, et al. PCOS in Adolescents—ongoing riddles in diagnosis and treatment. J Clin Med. 2023;12(3):1221.
11. Kaur I, Suri V, Rana SV, et al. Treatment pathways traversed by polycystic ovary syndrome (PCOS) patients: a mixed-method study. PLoS One. 2021; 16(8):e0255830.
12. Tolins ML, Rana JS, Lippert S, et al. Implementation and effectiveness of a physician-focused peer support program. PLoS One. 2023;18(11):e0292917.
13. Avery J, Ottey S, Morman R, et al. Polycystic ovary syndrome support groups and their role in awareness, advocacy and peer support: a systematic search and narrative review. Curr Opin Endocr Metabol Res. 2020;12:98-104.
14. Chung JE. Social networking in online support groups for health: how online social networking benefits patients. J Health Commun. 2014;19(6):639-59.
15. Teede HJ, Tay CT, Laven JJ, et al. Recommendations from the 2023 international evidence-based guideline for the assessment and management of polycystic ovary syndrome. Eur J Endocrinol. 2023;189(2):G43-64.